**S0-AXR-193**

ARE YOU WATCHING YOUR FAT INTAKE?
TRYING TO MAINTAIN A HEALTHY LIFESTYLE?

COOK WITH CONFIDENCE WITH
CORINNE T. NETZER'S
**COMPLETE BOOK OF FOOD COUNTS**
**COOKBOOK SERIES**
DON'T MISS . . .

### CRAB BITES

Everybody loves good crab cakes, but not everyone can abide by the concoction normally fried in globs of grease. Now with this recipe, you can enjoy them worry-free!
95 calories; 16.0 grams protein; 3.5 grams carbohydrates; 1.8 grams fat; 42.0 milligrams cholesterol; 450 milligrams sodium

### OVEN-FRIED HADDOCK WITH GARLIC-YOGURT CRUMB CRUST

A delicious, big-flaked white fish with a subtle sweetness, haddock is a hearty yet sophisticated dish . . . and a very low calorie one, too.
150 calories; 24.0 grams protein; 7.8 grams carbohydrates; 2.3 grams fat; 66.1 milligrams cholesterol; 170 milligrams sodium

### BUTTERFLY SHRIMP SAUTÉED WITH JALAPEÑOS

Bring a bit of the Southwest to your dining table, but look out gringos—these shrimp are big, juicy, and HOT!
150 calories; 24.0 grams protein; 7.0 grams carbohydrates; 2.9 grams fat; 173.0 milligrams cholesterol; 195 milligrams sodium

# 100 LOW FAT
# FISH AND
# SHELLFISH
# RECIPES

THE COMPLETE BOOK OF
FOOD COUNTS COOKBOOK SERIES

# 100 LOW FAT FISH AND SHELLFISH RECIPES

Corinne T. Netzer

A Dell Book

Published by
Dell Publishing
a division of
Bantam Doubleday Dell Publishing Group, Inc.
1540 Broadway
New York, New York 10036

ISBN: 0-440-22352-0

Printed in the United States of America

Published simultaneously in Canada

April 1997

10   9   8   7   6   5   4   3   2   1

OPM

# CONTENTS

# INTRODUCTION

Delicious! Delicious! Delicious! This is one of six books that comprise my Complete Book of Food Counts Cookbook Series—which also includes *100 Low Fat Pasta and Grain Recipes, 100 Low Fat Chicken and Turkey Recipes, 100 Low Fat Vegetable and Legume Recipes, 100 Low Fat Soup and Stew Recipes,* and *100 Low Fat Small Meal and Salad Recipes.* And all the recipes are *delicious*!

We are all aware of the need to reduce the fat in our diets, and ordinarily this would mean a sacrifice in taste. How many of us have had the misfortune to sample some very forgettable low fat dishes, where the overriding concern was only the fat content? It is my belief that no matter how "good" something is for you, you will not continue to eat it if it doesn't *taste* good, and this will almost certainly defeat your diet.

Every recipe in this book has been tested and sampled so that each dish is as good tasting as it is good for you. Low fat ingredients were not used automatically because they might fit or seemed right. Everything was tried out, because not all ingredients are interchangeable—and what might make sense in theory or at the drawing board may not please the palate.

Here you will find wonderful dishes—both plain and fancy—simple fare to eat and serve on a daily basis, and simply elegant fare that you will be proud to serve on any special occasion. Attention has been paid to the use of herbs and spices, but all the ingredients in these recipes can be found either in your cupboard or in the supermarket.

Good eating!

CTN

# A KEY TO COOKING FISH

Many cooks and food writers quote the Canadian rule when asked how to time the cooking of fish. The rule calls for eight to ten minutes per inch. While this is a good rule, it's not absolutely foolproof. A really thin fillet of fish might need less cooking, while a thick steak might require more.

Overcooking can result in a dry, tasteless dish, and the current fashion in trendy restaurants calls for fish that is slightly undercooked. Many professional chefs feel that fish should never be cooked to flakiness, and prefer fish that is translucent in the center. The result may be moist fish, but according to many health authorities rare fish is not always safe to eat, and they recommend eating fish that is thoroughly cooked.

What to do when faced with these pros and cons? The safest answer is to cook fish so that it is done, but not overdone. To achieve this, test the fish while it is being cooked—you can always return it to the skillet or broiler for further cooking, but you can't reverse an overdone fish.

Here are some simple ways to recognize a well-cooked fish: When grilling, broiling or sautéing, look for small drops of moisture that appear on the surface of the fish; when poaching remove fish from liquid when the fish flakes when tested with a fork; when cooking a whole fish pull on the dorsal fin, if it comes out easily, the fish is done.

No matter how you prefer your fish cooked, remember to always—*always*—start with the freshest fish you can find.

# STOCKS
# AND SAUCES
# FOR FISH

# LOW FAT CHICKEN STOCK

Chicken stock in fish recipes? The answer is a resounding Yes! Chicken stock is often more subtle and less assertive than fish stock. Fish stock, diluted or not, may sometimes compete with, rather than complement, fish dishes while chicken stock may strike the perfect balance of power.

For convenience, freeze one-cup portions of stock to use in recipes; it will keep for about a month. Or refrigerate the stock for up to one week.

2½ pounds chicken parts (backs, wings, necks)
10 cups water
½ cup dry white wine, optional
1 large onion, quartered
2 large carrots, coarsely chopped
2 large stalks celery, with tops, coarsely chopped
1 clove garlic, optional
1 bay leaf
10 whole peppercorns
8 sprigs fresh parsley
Salt to taste

1. Combine all ingredients in a soup pot and bring to a boil. Cover, reduce heat to very low, and simmer for about 3 hours. Skim stock as necessary. Remove from heat and let cool to room temperature.

2. Strain stock and discard solids or reserve for other use.

3. Cover and refrigerate stock for about 3 or 4 hours or until very well chilled.

4. Skim off hardened surface fat and discard. Stock is ready to be used or may be refrigerated or frozen in airtight containers for later use.

MAKES ABOUT 8 CUPS

Per 1 cup: 20 calories; 1.0 gram protein; 2.5 grams carbohydrates; .5 gram fat; .5 milligram cholesterol; 65 milligrams sodium (without salting).

# FISH STOCK

This basic fish stock can be used whenever a fish-accented broth is called for.

12 ounces fish parts (bones and heads from white-
     fleshed, non-oily fish, such as flounder, sole,
     whiting, etc.), gills removed
 7 cups water
 1 cup dry white wine
 1 carrot, halved
 2 stalks celery, halved
 1 small onion, halved
 1 tablespoon chopped fresh parsley
 1 bay leaf
   Salt and freshly ground pepper to taste

1. Combine all ingredients, except salt and pepper, in a soup pot and bring to a boil. Cover, reduce heat to low, and simmer for 20 minutes. Skim stock as necessary. Remove from heat and let cool slightly.

2. Strain stock and discard solids. Taste and add salt and pepper, if necessary. Use immediately or refrigerate or freeze in airtight containers for future use.

MAKES ABOUT 6 CUPS
Per 1 cup: 23 calories; 1.0 gram protein; 1.0 gram carbohydrates; .5 gram fat; .5 milligram cholesterol; 70 milligrams sodium (without salting).

# LIGHT ROUILLE

This garlic-hot pepper sauce is based on *rouille*, the sauce traditionally served with fish soup and bouillabaisse. The classic *rouille* calls for quantities of olive oil while this version keeps the oil to a minimum—the result is a richly flavored sauce low in fat.

1 medium potato, peeled and boiled
1/2 cup Low Fat Chicken Stock (page 3) or canned low
    sodium broth, heated to a simmer
2 teaspoons olive oil
1/4 teaspoon hot pepper sauce
1/4 cup chopped red bell pepper, blanched
4 cloves garlic, pressed
    Salt and freshly ground pepper to taste

1. Combine potato, stock, oil and hot pepper sauce in a mixing bowl. Mash until potato is completely free of lumps.

2. Add bell pepper and garlic to potato mixture and stir to blend thoroughly. Season to taste with salt and pepper.

MAKES ABOUT 1 CUP
Per 2 tablespoons: 25 calories; .5 gram protein; 3.5 grams carbohydrates; 1.2 grams fat; 0 milligrams cholesterol; 10 milligrams sodium (without salting).

# ALMOST AIOLI

*Aioli* is a marvelous garlicky mayonnaise that the French often use with steamed and broiled fish. They also add large spoons of *aioli* to fish soup for an added fillip. Here's a low calorie, low fat version of this wonderful sauce. Keep it in mind when serving cold shrimp and any simply prepared fish.

4 cloves garlic, quartered
1 slice white bread, broken into 4 pieces
2 tablespoons low fat (2%) milk
2 teaspoons Dijon mustard
1 cup low fat plain yogurt
Pinch salt, or to taste

1. Combine garlic, bread, milk, and mustard in a food processor and puree.

2. Spoon garlic mixture into a small bowl. Add yogurt gradually, stirring to blend. Season to taste. Cover and refrigerate for at least 1 hour to blend flavors before serving.

MAKES ABOUT 1¹/₂ CUPS
Per 2 tablespoons: 20 calories; 1.5 grams protein; 2.5 grams carbohydrates; .5 gram fat; 1 milligram cholesterol; 50 milligrams sodium (without salting).

# SALSA MEXICANA

Forget ordinary hot sauce when serving a shrimp cocktail, and ignore ketchup if you make hamburgers. Here's a spicy sauce that goes with fish or meat and can be used as a dip. Store in refrigerator for a week or more.

> 1 large onion, finely chopped
> 1 pound ripe tomatoes, peeled, seeded, and finely chopped
> 2 fresh jalapeño or serrano peppers, cored, seeded and minced (wear gloves), or 1 teaspoon red pepper flakes, or ½ cup canned, chopped green chilies, drained
> 1 clove garlic, pressed
> 1 tablespoon minced fresh cilantro
> Salt to taste

Combine all ingredients in a medium bowl. Mix thoroughly and allow flavors to blend for at least 1 hour before serving.

MAKES ABOUT 2 CUPS
Per 2 tablespoons: 12 calories; .4 gram protein; 2.5 grams carbohydrates; .1 gram fat; 0 milligrams cholesterol; 5 milligrams sodium (without salting).

# CUCUMBER SAUCE

This sauce is a nonfat yogurt/light sour cream variation of raita (a whole milk yogurt dish) that I
serve with cold poached fish, fish mousse, or terrine. I also like this light sauce with Indian or
other highly flavored cuisines.

    1 medium cucumber, peeled, seeded, and quartered
    1 small onion, quartered
    ¼ cup packed fresh dill weed
    1 cup nonfat plain yogurt
    ½ cup light sour cream

Place cucumber, onion, and dill weed in a food
processor and chop coarsely. Add yogurt and sour
cream and continue processing until ingredients are
just combined. Spoon sauce into a small bowl and
chill before serving.

MAKES ABOUT 2 CUPS
Per ¼ cup: 45 calories; 3.0 grams protein; 5.2 grams carbohydrates; 1.4 grams fat; 1.7 milligrams cholesterol; 45
milligrams sodium (without salting).

# GREEN SAUCE WITH SHALLOTS

I've trimmed the fat of the classic Spanish *salsa verde* by drastically reducing the amount of olive oil used in the original. Thick and tangy, my adaptation animates any plain fish—whether broiled, grilled, steamed, or poached. It's best at room temperature.

*1½ cups trimmed fresh Italian parsley*
  *1 cup trimmed fresh watercress*
  *2 large shallots, chopped*
  *1 tablespoon fresh tarragon or 1 teaspoon dried*
    *Juice of 1 large lemon*
    *Salt and freshly ground pepper to taste*
*1½ tablespoons olive oil*

Combine all ingredients, except olive oil, in a food processor and process briefly, until greens are coarsely chopped. With machine running, add oil in a slow, steady stream and process until ingredients are well blended.

MAKES ABOUT 1½ CUPS
Per 2 tablespoons: 18 calories; 1.0 gram protein; 1.0 gram carbohydrates; 1.0 gram fat; 0 milligrams cholesterol; 5 milligrams sodium (without salting).

# TOMATO-GINGER MARINADE AND GRILLING SAUCE

This light sauce will flesh out the flavor of most high fat or moderately fatty fish, including salmon, tuna, mackerel, sardines, and trout. The aromatic ginger-tomato combination lends an alluring touch to the fish as well as adding moisture and protection.

*1 cup canned no-salt-added tomato sauce*
*3 tablespoons red wine vinegar*
*1 tablespoon Worcestershire sauce*
*1 small onion, finely minced*
*1 large clove garlic, pressed*
*1 tablespoon finely minced peeled ginger root, or to taste*
*1 teaspoon dry mustard*
*2 tablespoons olive oil*
*Salt and freshly ground pepper to taste*
*2 teaspoons sugar or to taste, optional*

Combine all ingredients, except salt, pepper, and sugar, in a blender or large jar with a tight-fitting lid and mix until thoroughly blended. Taste and add salt, pepper and sugar, if desired. Let stand at least 1 hour before using to blend flavors.

Per ¼ cup serving: 65 calories; 1.0 gram protein; 4.5 grams carbohydrates; 4.7 grams fat; 0 milligrams cholesterol; 35 milligrams sodium (without salting).

# REMOULADE SAUCE

This classic French sauce is traditionally made with heaps of rich mayonnaise. As one might expect, Remoulade is usually a very high fat, high calorie affair (about 100 calories and 14 grams fat per tablespoon!), while my streamlined version, containing low fat yogurt instead of mayonnaise, is just as rich in flavor.

This versatile sauce is perfect with fish cakes and chilled steamed clams or mussels, as a spread on sandwiches, and as a superb dressing for seafood salad. Refrigerate in an airtight container for up to a week.

1 cup low fat plain yogurt
1 tablespoon Dijon mustard
2 cloves garlic, chopped
3 anchovy fillets, rinsed and diced
1/4 cup chopped fresh Italian parsley
2 tablespoons fresh tarragon or 1 tablespoon dried
1 tablespoon balsamic vinegar
1 tablespoon fresh lemon juice
3 small cornichons, chopped
2 tablespoons small capers, rinsed and drained
1 1/2 tablespoons olive oil
    Salt and freshly ground pepper to taste

1. Combine all ingredients, except capers, oil, salt and pepper, in a food processor and process very

briefly. With machine running, add oil in a slow, steady stream.

2. Transfer to a small mixing bowl and stir in capers. Taste and season, if necessary, with salt and pepper.

<small>MAKES ABOUT</small> 1¾ <small>CUPS</small>
Per 2 tablespoons: 30 calories; 1.5 grams protein; 2.0 grams carbohydrates; 1.7 grams fat; 1 milligram cholesterol; 120 milligrams sodium (without salting).

# SOUPS, STEWS, AND CHOWDERS

# ASIAN RICE AND SALMON SOUP

Because the salmon will cook in the bowl, slicing it as thinly as possible is a must for this dish. One way to accomplish this is by partially freezing the fish then using a very sharp knife. An easier way is to ask your fishmonger to do it for you.

1/2 pound salmon fillets, skin removed, very thinly sliced (as for sushi or sashimi)
2 teaspoons low sodium soy sauce
3 teaspoons vegetable oil
1 tablespoon grated peeled ginger
4 scallions, white and tender greens, minced
1/4 cup rice
5 cups Fish Stock (page 5)
1 tablespoon flavored rice wine vinegar
1/2 teaspoon hot pepper sauce
2 tablespoons finely chopped fresh basil leaves

1. Place salmon in a shallow dish. Combine soy sauce with 1 teaspoon of the oil. Mix and spoon over salmon. Refrigerate for 30 minutes, turning salmon twice in marinade.

2. Heat remaining 2 teaspoons oil in a soup pot. Add ginger and scallions, and cook, stirring, for 30 seconds. Add rice and stock. Cover and bring to a boil. Stir, reduce heat to low, and simmer for 15 to 20 minutes or until the rice is tender.

3. Add rice wine vinegar and hot pepper sauce to soup and stir.

4. Divide salmon slices among 4 heated soup bowls. Bring soup to a rolling boil then ladle it over salmon in bowls—the hot soup will cook the thinly sliced salmon. Garnish with chopped basil and serve.

SERVES 4

Per serving: 140 calories; 7.0 grams protein; 18.2 grams carbohydrates; 4.5 grams fat (1.6 grams fat from fish); 14 milligrams cholesterol; 195 milligrams sodium (without salting).

# SOUP OF MUSSELS
# WITH SHALLOTS AND WINE

Excellent as a summer's lunch, it also makes a lovely first or main course any time of the year.

  2 teaspoons olive oil
 10 shallots, chopped
  1 carrot, thinly sliced
  1 stalk celery, thinly sliced
 $1/2$ cup chopped fresh dill weed
  1 teaspoon dried thyme
 $1/2$ teaspoon hot red pepper flakes or to taste
  4 cups Fish Stock (page 5), Low Fat Chicken Stock
       (page 3), or canned low sodium broth
  1 cup dry white wine
  2 dozen mussels, scrubbed, debearded, and rinsed
       Salt and freshly ground pepper to taste

1. Heat oil in a soup pot. Add all ingredients except mussels, salt, and pepper. Cover and bring to a simmer. Cook over low heat, stirring frequently, for 3 minutes.

2. Add mussels, raise heat to medium, cover again, and cook for 5 to 6 minutes, or until shells have opened. Discard any mussels that have not opened.

3. Taste to adjust seasoning and add salt and pepper if necessary. Ladle mussels and soup into 4 deep bowls and serve.

Serves 4

Per serving: 230 calories; 17.0 grams protein; 28.5 grams carbohydrates; 5.5 grams fat (3.0 grams fat from fish); 31 milligrams cholesterol; 415 milligrams sodium (without salting).

# FISH SOUP PROVENÇAL

I could live on this delicious soup and never be "nutritionally challenged." Once you get the hang of the proportions of veggies to fish, liquid, and seasonings, go ahead and improvise! You may wish to add or substitute other sturdy fish, or experiment with other spices.

The Light Rouille sauce adds a tasty and elegant touch, but the soup can also be enjoyed without it.

*½ cup Low Fat Chicken Stock (page 3) or canned low sodium broth*

*1 teaspoon olive oil*

*1 large onion, chopped*

*2 cloves garlic, halved*

*2 green bell peppers, chopped*

*1 carrot, chopped*

*1 stalk celery, chopped*

*2 ripe tomatoes, peeled and chopped, with juice*

*¾ pound assorted fish fillets (cod, halibut, haddock, bass), cubed*

*½ teaspoon herbes de Provence or combination of dried thyme, rosemary, marjoram, sage*

*1 1-inch piece dried orange peel*

*½ cup dry white wine or dry vermouth*

*4 cups water*

*Salt and freshly ground pepper to taste*

*½ cup Light Rouille (page 6), optional*

1. Combine stock and oil in a soup pot and heat. Add onion, garlic, bell pepper, carrot and celery and cook over low heat, stirring occasionally, for 15 minutes.

2. Add all remaining ingredients, except Light Rouille. Cover and simmer over low heat, stirring occasionally, for 20 minutes.

3. Transfer contents of pot to a food processor and puree. You may have to do this in two or more steps.

4. Return pureed soup to pot and heat to a simmer. Taste and adjust seasonings, if necessary. Serve in large heated bowls, and offer the Light Rouille sauce on the side.

SERVES 4

Per serving: 145 calories; 17.0 grams protein; 14.8 grams carbohydrates; 2.1 grams fat (.6 gram fat from fish); 36 milligrams cholesterol; 80 milligrams sodium (without salting).

# CANTONESE FISH BALL SOUP

This recipe does double duty. I sometimes just serve the fish balls, accompanied by a dipping sauce, as an appetizer or party offering.

*¾ pound fish fillets (flounder, sole, cod, or bass), cut into chunks*
*2 egg whites*
*⅓ cup water*
*¼ teaspoon sugar*
*1 teaspoon hot pepper sauce or to taste*
*1 tablespoon cornstarch*
*2 teaspoons vegetable oil*
*5 cups Low Fat Chicken Stock (page 3) or canned low sodium broth*
*2 scallions, sliced*
*¼ cup fresh bean sprouts*
*6 fresh water chestnuts, sliced, or ¼ cup canned sliced water chestnuts*

1. Bring about 2 quarts of water to a boil in a large pot.

2. Meanwhile, place fish fillets in a food processor. Add egg whites, water, sugar, hot pepper sauce, cornstarch, and vegetable oil. Process until mixture is smoothly pureed.

3. Form fish mixture into 1-inch balls and drop into boiling water. Reduce heat and allow fish balls

to simmer for 10 minutes. Remove fish balls from water and drain.

4. Heat stock or broth in a soup pot. Add fish balls, bring broth to a simmer and cook for 10 minutes. Transfer fish balls and broth to a heated tureen or large soup bowls. Garnish each serving with equal amounts of scallion, bean sprouts, and water chestnuts.

SERVES 4

Per serving: 155 calories; 18.0 grams protein; 12.5 grams carbohydrates; 3.6 grams fat (.6 gram fat from fish); 36 milligrams cholesterol; 160 milligrams sodium (without salting).

# SALMON AND
# ARTICHOKE HEARTS
# IN CREAMY BROTH

Think of this dense and delicious soup as a kind of fat-curbed vichyssoise and you've got an idea of the concept behind this dish. I've omitted the cream and substituted rich-tasting low fat evaporated milk, and bolstered the flavor by adding hearts of artichoke, peas, and a goodly amount of salmon. In fact, this soup is so hearty, it can be served as a main course!

    1 tablespoon vegetable or olive oil
    3 leeks, white and tender greens, well-rinsed and
        finely chopped
    1 clove garlic, minced
    3 cups Low Fat Chicken Stock (page 3) or canned low
        sodium broth
    2 large potatoes, peeled and cubed
        Salt and freshly ground pepper to taste
    2 cups cooked quartered artichoke hearts, fresh,
        frozen, or canned
    3/4 pound salmon fillets, skin removed, cut into pieces
    1 cup fresh or frozen and thawed green peas
    1/2 cup evaporated low fat milk
    2 tablespoons minced fresh chives or scallion greens

    1. Heat oil in a soup pot. Add leeks and garlic and cook, stirring, over medium heat for 3 minutes

or until leeks are just tender. Do not let leeks brown.

2. Add stock to pot and bring to a simmer. Add potatoes and salt and pepper to taste. Reduce heat to low, cover, and simmer gently for 10 minutes, stirring occasionally. Add artichoke hearts and simmer an additional 10 minutes.

3. Add salmon and peas to pot and simmer, uncovered, for 5 to 8 minutes or until salmon is just cooked through.

4. Add milk and simmer, stirring, for 1 minute or until ingredients are thoroughly heated and blended. Transfer to heated bowls, sprinkle with chives or scallion greens, and serve.

SERVES 4

Per serving: 330 calories; 18.0 grams protein; 47.5 grams carbohydrates; 7.5 grams fat (2.4 grams fat from fish); 21 milligrams cholesterol; 205 milligrams sodium (without salting).

# CALICO CHOWDER
# WITH ESCAROLE AND ORZO

Calicos are members of the scallop family. Originating in southern waters, they are smaller and more plentiful than the more delicately flavored—and much more expensive—bay scallop. Their more pronounced flavor make calicos perfect in this sturdy, nutritious chowder. Try this with oyster crackers.

1 teaspoon olive oil
1 medium head escarole lettuce, well-rinsed, drained, and cut into 2-inch pieces
5 cups Low Fat Chicken Stock (page 3) or canned low sodium broth
3/4 pound calico scallops
1/2 cup orzo, acini di pepe, or other small pasta
1/4 cup minced red bell pepper
Salt and freshly ground pepper to taste

1. Heat oil in a soup pot. Add escarole and cook over medium-high heat, stirring, for 2 minutes. Add stock, reduce heat to very low, cover, and simmer for about 10 minutes or until escarole is tender.

2. Raise heat to medium and bring stock to a simmer. Add calicos and orzo, cover, and cook for about 5 minutes or until pasta is al dente and calicos are cooked through.

3. Add bell pepper and salt and pepper to taste.

Stir for 1 minute. Remove from heat, ladle into heated soup bowls, and serve.

SERVES 4

Per serving: 245 calories; 20.2 grams protein; 34.5 grams carbohydrates; 3.0 grams fat (.7 gram fat from fish); 29 milligrams cholesterol; 250 milligrams sodium (without salting).

# MANHATTAN CLAM CHOWDER
# WITH FRESH BASIL

Does anyone know why clam chowder made with tomatoes is called Manhattan Clam Chowder, while chowder made with milk or cream is called New England Clam Chowder? I've never gotten a satisfactory answer to that question, but here is a satisfying recipe for the tomato-based variety of chowder. Fresh basil adds compatible character.

> 2 dozen cherrystone or littleneck clams, scrubbed and
>     rinsed
> 1 cup cold water
> 2 teaspoons olive oil
> 1 medium onion, chopped
> 2 stalks celery, thinly sliced
> 1 clove garlic, pressed
> 1 carrot, thinly sliced
> 1 bay leaf
> 2 medium potatoes, peeled and cubed
> 2 ripe plum tomatoes, coarsely chopped
> 1 cup low sodium tomato juice
> 4 cups Fish Stock (page 5), Low Fat Chicken Stock
>     (page 3), or canned low sodium broth
> 2 tablespoons finely minced fresh basil or parsley
>     Salt and freshly ground pepper to taste

1. Place clams in a soup pot and add water. Cover and steam over high heat for about 8 minutes or

until shells have opened. Remove clams from liquid and discard any clams that have not opened. Set aside clams to cool. Strain cooking liquid and reserve.

2. Heat oil in the soup pot. Add onion, celery, garlic, carrot, and bay leaf. Cook, uncovered, over low heat, stirring occasionally, for 5 minutes.

3. Add reserved cooking liquid from clams, and all remaining ingredients, except clams, basil, and salt and pepper, to pot. Cover and bring to a simmer. Cook for about 20 minutes or until potatoes are tender.

4. Remove clams from shells and chop coarsely. Add clams to pot, along with basil and salt and pepper to taste. Stir to combine and cook an additional minute or until ingredients are simmering. Remove bay leaf. Transfer soup to a heated tureen or individual bowls and serve.

SERVES 4

Per serving: 175 calories; 10.5 grams protein; 26.5 grams carbohydrates; 3.5 grams fat (.9 gram fat from fish); 18 milligrams cholesterol; 135 milligrams sodium (without salting).

# SHRIMP-TOMATO BISQUE WITH CORIANDER

"Bisque" is a thick, rich soup usually containing pureed seafood and cream. This slimmed-down version adds the zing of cayenne to the mix and reduces the fat count to a more acceptable level.

I like to serve this with homemade melba toast, oven-toasted pita triangle, matzo crackers, or heated Indian paratha (without the clarified butter).

    ½ pound medium shrimp, rinsed
  1½ tablespoons margarine
    1 medium onion, coarsely chopped
    1 large stalk celery, coarsely chopped
    4 ripe tomatoes, chopped, with juice
    2 tablespoons no-salt-added tomato paste
    1 teaspoon ground coriander
    ¼ teaspoon cayenne or to taste
    3 cups Fish Stock (page 5), Low Fat Chicken Stock
        (page 3), or canned low sodium broth
    ½ cup dry white wine
    1 tablespoon fine flour
    ½ cup low fat (2%) milk
      Salt to taste
    2 tablespoons minced fresh cilantro or chopped chives

1. Peel and devein shrimp, reserving shells. Dice all but 4 of the shrimp and set aside.

2. Heat margarine in a nonstick soup pot. Add shrimp shells and stir over medium heat for about 1 minute or until shells are pink. Using a slotted spoon, remove and discard shells.

3. Add onion and celery to pot with margarine and cook over low heat, stirring frequently, for 3 minutes or until just tender.

4. Add diced shrimp, tomatoes, tomato paste, coriander and cayenne to pot and stir to combine. Cook at a slow simmer for 5 minutes. Add stock or broth and wine and bring to boil. Lower heat and simmer gently, stirring occasionally, for 10 minutes.

5. Strain liquid into another pot and place solids into a food processor. Bring liquid to a simmer and process solids until smoothly pureed. Add pureed solids and stir until well-blended and simmering.

6. Stir flour with milk in a small bowl and add to pot. Simmer, stirring, until thickened. Taste and add salt and adjust seasonings if needed.

7. Transfer soup to heated bowls. Add a shrimp to each bowl, sprinkle with cilantro or chives, and serve.

SERVES 4

Per serving: 190 calories; 15.0 grams protein; 19.0 grams carbohydrates; 6.0 grams fat (1.2 grams fat from fish); 89 milligrams cholesterol; 220 milligrams sodium (without salting).

# CREAMY SQUASH
# AND OYSTER SOUP

This is my creamless variation on a simple oyster stew. The squash and stock add texture and taste and make this soup a stunning opener for any meal.

> 1 Hubbard squash (about 1¼ pounds), peeled, seeded
>     and cut into 1-inch cubes
> 4 cups Low Fat Chicken Stock (page 3) or canned low
>     sodium broth
> ¼ cup dry sherry (not cooking wine)
> 1 teaspoon mild paprika, plus 1 teaspoon for garnish
> 1 tablespoon cornstarch
> 1 cup evaporated low fat milk
> ½ pound or ½ pint shucked oysters, with its liquor
>     Salt to taste

1. Combine squash and stock or broth, sherry, and 1 teaspoon paprika in a soup pot. Bring to a boil, then reduce heat to low, cover, and simmer gently, stirring occasionally, for about 45 minutes or until squash is very tender. This soup should be a little lumpy so mash squash against the pot with a wooden spoon if necessary.

2. Dissolve cornstarch in milk in a small bowl and add to soup. Stir, uncovered, over medium-high heat until soup starts to simmer. Add oysters with liquor and continue to cook, stirring, long enough

for edges of the oysters to curl and soup to be thoroughly heated.

3. Taste and add salt, if desired. Transfer soup to a heated tureen or individual bowls, sprinkle with remaining paprika, and serve.

SERVES 4
Per serving: 170 calories; 10.8 grams protein; 22.5 grams carbohydrates; 3.9 grams fat (1.4 grams fat from fish); 36 milligrams cholesterol; 200 milligrams sodium (without salting).

# FISH CHOWDER SAN FRANCISCO (CIOPPINO)

Italian immigrants who settled in San Francisco are credited with creating "cioppino" (pronounced chuh-PEE-noh), an absolutely superb stew made with tomatoes and a variety of just-caught fish and shellfish.

This recipe is adapted from the best of San Francisco's Fisherman's Wharf. If you live near that coast, use Pacific snapper, ling cod, and Dungeness crab when preparing this dish. If you're an Easterner buy red snapper, cod, or halibut. Finally, Alaska king crab legs can be bought just about anywhere in the country. The key factor in making this or any fish and shellfish dish successfully is to prepare it with the freshest ingredients you can find.

    1 tablespoon olive oil
    1 medium onion, chopped
    2 cloves garlic, pressed
    4 large tomatoes, peeled and chopped, with juice
    1 can (2 ounces) no-salt-added tomato paste
    1 medium green bell pepper, chopped
    1/2 teaspoon dried oregano
    6 fresh basil leaves, chopped, or 1/2 teaspoon dried
        basil
    1 bay leaf

1/4 teaspoon hot red pepper flakes or to taste
1 cup dry red wine
2 cups water
1/2 pound fish fillets (Pacific or red snapper, ling cod,
  Eastern cod, halibut, or combination)
1/4 pound bay scallops or quartered sea scallops
6 large shrimp, shelled and deveined
6 clams, scrubbed
1 Dungeness crab, cracked, or 1/2 pound frozen Alaska
  King crab legs, thawed
Salt and freshly ground pepper to taste

1. Heat oil in a soup pot or Dutch oven. Add onion and garlic and cook, stirring, for 3 minutes, or until onion is translucent. Add tomatoes, tomato paste, and a tomato-paste canful of water and cook, stirring, for an additional minute or until ingredients are blended.

2. Add green pepper, seasonings, wine, and water to pot and stir to combine. Cover, and simmer over low heat for 30 minutes.

3. Cut fish fillets into large pieces and add to pot. Cook for 1 minute. Raise heat, add shellfish and cook, covered, stirring occasionally, for 5 to 7 minutes or until fish is cooked through and clams have opened. Remove bay leaf. Taste and adjust seasonings or add salt and pepper and serve.

Per serving: 150 calories; 15.5 grams protein; 11.5 grams carbohydrates; 3.6 grams fat (1.0 gram fat from fish); 56 milligrams cholesterol; 170 milligrams sodium (without salting).

# SOUTHWESTERN SEAFOOD STEW WITH BEANS

This recipe would be equally at home in Santa Fe, Topeka, or Staten Island. The stew combines a variety of diverse ingredients to create a dish that is pleasing to both the palate and the eye.

Just recently, while fiddling around in the kitchen, I substituted a large sweet potato, diced into ½-inch cubes, for the beans with excellent results—proving that no recipe is carved in stone . . . the possibilities are endless!

    1 tablespoon olive oil
    1 medium zucchini, diced
    1 large onion, diced
    1 large stalk celery, chopped
    2 cloves garlic, minced
    1 medium red bell pepper, trimmed, seeded, and diced
    1 medium green bell pepper, trimmed, seeded, and
        diced
    2 small jalapeño peppers, seeded and diced
    5 ripe tomatoes, chopped, with juice
    1 cup canned no-salt-added tomato sauce
    1 tablespoon hot or mild chili powder or to taste
    1 teaspoon ground cumin
    1 teaspoon dried oregano
    ½ cup chopped fresh cilantro or flat-leaf parsley
    2 cups cooked or canned (no-salt added or rinsed) red
        kidney beans

*¹/₄ pound small or medium shrimp, shelled and
    deveined*
*¹/₂ pound fish fillets (sole, flounder, or cod), cut into
    1-inch pieces*
*2 tablespoons fresh lemon juice*
*¹/₂ pound bay scallops or quartered sea scallops, rinsed*
*¹/₂ cup finely minced scallions*

1. Heat oil in a soup pot. Add zucchini, onion, celery, garlic, bell peppers, and jalapeños and cook over medium low heat, stirring frequently, for about 8 minutes or until vegetables are tender.

2. Add tomatoes, tomato sauce, chili powder, cumin, oregano, and cilantro. Stir over low heat until thoroughly combined. Add beans and let simmer gently for 5 minutes.

3. Add shrimp, fish fillets, and lemon juice to pot. Stir gently to combine ingredients and simmer over medium heat for 2 minutes. Add scallops and simmer for an additional 3 to 5 minutes or until all the fish is cooked through.

4. Transfer to a heated tureen, a deep platter, or individual bowls, sprinkle with scallions, and serve.

SERVES 6
Per serving: 240 calories; 24.0 grams protein; 27.5 grams carbohydrates; 4.5 grams fat (.9 gram fat from fish); 57 milligrams cholesterol; 155 milligrams sodium (without salting).

# SCROD AND VEGETABLE STEW

Inspired by the wonderful flavors beloved by the people of the Mediterranean region, I pay homage with this delicious stew. Easy to prepare and ready to present in no time at all, it's the kind of last-minute meal I rely on when unexpected guests arrive at my door. A fast walk to my fish store or supermarket will assure me of getting the freshest fish possible. The rest of the ingredients are almost always available in my pantry, refrigerator, or freezer.

  1 tablespoon olive oil
  1 onion, halved and thinly sliced
  2 stalks celery, chopped
  2 cloves garlic, minced
  1/4 cup coarsely chopped fresh flat-leaf parsley
  1 bay leaf
  1/2 teaspoon each: dried thyme and marjoram
  2 cups Fish Stock (page 5) or water
  2 large potatoes, peeled and cut into 1-inch cubes
  2 cups chopped fresh tomatoes with juice, or canned
      no-salt-added tomatoes
    Salt and freshly ground pepper to taste
    Pinch cayenne or to taste, optional
  1/3 pound green beans, trimmed and cut into 1/2-inch
      pieces
  3/4 pound scrod, cod, or white fish fillets

1. Heat oil in a nonstick soup pot. Add onion and celery and cook over low heat, stirring frequently, for 5 minutes. Stir in garlic, parsley, bay leaf, thyme, and marjoram. Cover and simmer gently for 5 minutes.

2. Raise heat to medium. Add stock or water and potatoes and cook, covered, for 10 minutes. Stir in tomatoes, salt and pepper, and cayenne, if desired. Reduce heat to low and cook for an additional 10 minutes.

3. Add green beans and place fish fillets over vegetables in pot. Cover, and simmer gently for about 8 minutes or until fish is just cooked through. Remove cover and raise heat to medium. Stir gently, breaking up fish into bite-size pieces, and let simmer for 5 minutes.

4. Remove bay leaf, ladle into heated bowls, and serve.

SERVES 6

Per serving: 150 calories; 12.5 grams protein; 18.5 grams carbohydrates; 3.2 grams fat (.5 gram fat from fish); 24 milligrams cholesterol; 75 milligrams sodium (without salting).

# CHILLED LOBSTER
# AND YOGURT SOUP

Carrots add color and sweetness to this delightful summer soup. Crabmeat can be substituted for the lobster.

   1 tablespoon margarine
   1 onion, chopped
   4 carrots, diced
   3 cups Low Fat Chicken Stock (page 3) or canned low
      sodium broth
 $^1/_2$ cup dry white wine
   1 tablespoon fine flour
      Salt to taste
 $^1/_2$ teaspoon ground cardamom
 $^1/_2$ teaspoon paprika or to taste
   1 cup low fat plain yogurt
 $^1/_2$ pound cooked lobster meat, shredded
      Paprika for garnish

1. Heat margarine in a nonstick skillet or soup pot. Add onion and carrots and cook, stirring, over low heat for 5 minutes. Add stock and wine and bring to a boil. Reduce heat to low and simmer gently for 10 minutes or until carrots are tender.

2. Using a slotted spoon, transfer carrots and onions to a food processor and process until vegetables are pureed.

3. Return pureed vegetables to liquid in skillet.

Add flour, salt, cardamom, and paprika and cook over medium heat, stirring, for 1 minute or until thoroughly blended and slightly thickened. Remove from heat and let cool slightly.

4. In a tureen or mixing bowl, combine contents of skillet with yogurt and stir to blend. Add lobster meat and blend thoroughly. Cover and refrigerate for 30 minutes to 1 hour or until chilled. Stir and serve in tureen or individual bowls, sprinkled with paprika.

SERVES 4

Per serving: 195 calories; 16.5 grams protein; 22.0 grams carbohydrates; 4.5 grams fat (.9 gram fat from fish); 45 milligrams cholesterol; 350 milligrams sodium (without salting).

# APPETIZERS
# AND
# SALADS

# FLOUNDER
# AND VEGETABLE TERRINE

When you cut into this lovely terrine with its layers of fish, delicious low fat, coriander-scented custard, and colorful vegetable mixture, your guests will be rewarded with a highly edible slice of still-life.

  *Vegetable oil cooking spray*
  *Egg substitute equal to 2 whole eggs*
  *1 small onion, halved*
  *4 ounces nonfat plain yogurt*
  *4 ounces low fat cottage cheese*
  *¼ teaspoon coriander seeds*
  *1 pound thinly sliced flounder fillets*
  *1 cup shredded carrots*
  *1 cup chopped broccoli florets*

1. Preheat oven to 350° F. Lightly coat a nonstick 6-cup terrine or loaf pan with vegetable spray and set aside.

2. Combine egg substitute, onion, yogurt, cottage cheese, and coriander seeds in a food processor and blend thoroughly.

3. Place half of fish fillets in reserved terrine or loaf pan. Spoon egg-yogurt mixture on top of fish and smooth to even out.

4. Combine carrots and broccoli and spoon over egg-yogurt mixture. Top with remaining fish slices

and cover with foil. Bake for 45 minutes. Let cool slightly, then transfer to a platter and serve.

SERVES 6

Per serving: 125 calories; 20.5 grams protein; 6.0 grams carbohydrates; 2.1 grams fat (.9 gram fat from fish); 39 milligrams cholesterol; 180 milligrams sodium (without salting).

# MOUSSE OF SOLE
# WITH CUCUMBER SAUCE

Here is a lighter-than-air dish that's also light on the fat and calories. Deceptively easy to prepare, it's always perfect fare for your crowd on a sultry summer's day. The Cucumber Sauce adds contrasting color and taste.

1½ pounds sole fillets
  1 cup low fat (2%) milk
  1 small onion, halved
  2 tablespoons all-purpose flour
    Egg substitute equal to 2 whole eggs
  2 egg whites, lightly beaten
    Salt and freshly ground pepper (preferably white) to
      taste
  ¼ cup packed fresh parsley
  ¼ cup packed fresh dill weed
  1 cup Cucumber Sauce (page 9)

1. Pour water into the bottom of a steamer. Place fish on steaming rack and cover. Bring water to a boil and steam for about 6 minutes or until fish flakes when tested with a fork. Remove fish from steamer and allow to cool.

2. Preheat oven to 400° F.

3. Cut fish into large pieces and combine with milk, onion, flour, egg substitute and whites, and salt and pepper in a food processor. Process until

mixture is smooth. Add parsley and dill and process only until incorporated into mixture.

4. Spoon mousse into a 6-cup nonstick loaf pan or ring mold and bake for 50 to 60 minutes or until top is brown and puffy and a knife inserted close to the center comes out clean. Let cool slightly. Slice and serve warm with Cucumber Sauce on the side.

SERVES 8
Per serving: 160 calories; 23.2 grams protein; 10.0 grams carbohydrates; 3.0 grams fat (1.0 gram fat from fish); 45 milligrams cholesterol; 160 milligrams sodium (without salting).

# SALMON-STUFFED ENDIVE

The felicitous combination of salmon with my low fat Cucumber Sauce is so good, I've been known to scarf down far more of these divine nibbles than my agreed-upon allotment.

This mixture can also be used as a filler for celery, cherry tomatoes, snow peas, as a dip for crudités, or—if the spirit moves you—as a spread on toasted bagels.

*½ pound salmon fillets*
*1 cup Cucumber Sauce (page 9)*
*  Salt and freshly ground pepper to taste*
*2 heads Belgian endive, rinsed and separated into*
*  leaves*

1. Pour water into the bottom of steamer. Place salmon on steaming rack and cover. Bring water to a boil and steam for 4 to 5 minutes, or until fish is cooked. Remove from steamer and allow to cool.

2. Remove skin, if any, from salmon and refrigerate for 1 hour.

3. Place salmon and ¼ cup of Cucumber Sauce in a food processor and process until just blended. Transfer to a medium mixing bowl and add remaining Cucumber Sauce. Mix thoroughly and season to taste with salt and pepper.

4. Using a small spoon, fill endive leaves with

salmon mixture and arrange on a platter before serving.

SERVES 4

Per serving: 125 calories; 11.0 grams protein; 13.5 grams carbohydrates; 3.4 grams fat (1.6 grams fat from fish); 14 milligrams cholesterol; 115 milligrams sodium (without salting).

# SHRIMP AND CANNELLINI BEANS BALSAMIC

Use regular white or great northern beans in place of cannellini beans, if desired. Best when served at room temperature or slightly chilled.

> *½ pound small or medium shrimp, rinsed, shelled, and deveined*
> *2 cups cooked cannellini (white kidney) beans, or canned (no-salt-added or well-rinsed and drained)*
> *6 scallions, whites and tender greens, chopped*
> *1 small red bell pepper, trimmed and minced*
> *¼ cup chopped fresh basil or Italian parsley*
> *¼ cup Low Fat Chicken Stock (page 3) or canned low sodium broth*
> *2 tablespoons balsamic vinegar*
> *1 tablespoon white wine vinegar*
> *1 tablespoon olive oil*
> *Salt and freshly ground pepper to taste*

1. Cook shrimp in a small saucepan full of boiling water for about 5 minutes or until shrimp turn pink and are cooked through. Drain and set aside to cool.

2. In a large bowl, combine beans with scallions, bell pepper, and basil. Add shrimp (cut medium shrimp in half) and toss gently to avoid breaking beans.

3. Combine remaining ingredients in a small bowl

and blend thoroughly. Add to bean-shrimp mixture
and toss gently to coat ingredients.

SERVES 6
Per serving: 130 calories; 12.5 grams protein; 12.5 grams
carbohydrates; 3.5 grams fat (.7 gram fat from fish); 58
milligrams cholesterol; 60 milligrams sodium (without
salting).

# SALAD OF BROILED SALMON WITH ZUCCHINI

Ritzy, glitzy, and kind to the arteries, this salad makes an excellent first course or light lunch or dinner. The balsamic vinaigrette, with its sweet pungency, is used to brush on the fish and zucchini and in the dressing for the completed dish.

 1 tablespoon olive oil
 2 tablespoons balsamic vinegar
 $^1/_2$ teaspoon fresh lemon juice
 $^1/_4$ teaspoon Dijon mustard
    Salt and freshly ground pepper to taste
 1 pound salmon fillets
 2 medium zucchini, each cut into $^1/_2$-inch slices
 1 head Boston or Bibb lettuce, rinsed and separated
    into leaves
12 small cherry tomatoes
 1 tablespoon minced fresh chives

1. Preheat broiler to high.

2. Combine oil, vinegar, lemon juice, mustard, and salt and pepper in a small jar with a tight-fitting lid. Close jar and shake until ingredients are thoroughly blended.

3. Place salmon and zucchini on a shallow nonstick broiler pan. Brush with oil-vinegar dressing and broil for 3 minutes. Turn salmon and zucchini, brush with dressing and broil for an additional 3

minutes, or until salmon and zucchini are cooked. Remove from broiler and allow to cool.

4. Combine lettuce, tomatoes, and chives in a bowl. Add remaining dressing and toss. Arrange lettuce mixture on salad plates. Cut salmon into 4 pieces and place on lettuce. Place zucchini slices around salmon and serve.

SERVES 4

Per serving: 135 calories; 11.5 grams protein; 6.0 grams carbohydrates; 7.0 grams fat (3.2 grams fat from fish); 28 milligrams cholesterol; 40 milligrams sodium (without salting).

# CRAB BITES

Everybody loves good crab cakes. But not everyone's body can abide by the concoction normally fried in globs of grease. My little crab "bites" combine delectable crabmeat with onion, egg substitute, low fat milk, mustard, hot red pepper sauce, and bread crumbs, which then get baked to a golden turn.

This is very good served with my Remoulade Sauce.

*Vegetable oil cooking spray*
*1 pound cooked crabmeat, cartilage removed*
*1 small onion*
*Egg substitute equal to 1 egg*
*1/4 cup low fat (2%) milk*
*1 teaspoon dry mustard*
*1/4 teaspoon hot pepper sauce*
*1/2 cup bread crumbs, made from 1 slice dry firm white bread (approximate)*
*1 cup Remoulade Sauce (page 13), optional*

1. Preheat oven to 400° F. Coat a shallow nonstick baking pan with cooking spray and set aside.

2. Combine crabmeat, onion, egg substitute, milk, mustard, and hot pepper sauce in a food processor. Process until thoroughly pureed. Add bread crumbs gradually until mixture forms a soft ball.

3. Form crabmeat mixture into small 1 1/2-inch

balls, adding more bread crumbs if necessary to hold crab mixture together. Arrange crab balls on reserved baking pan and bake for 15 to 20 minutes, turning once, or until lightly browned and crisp.

4. Transfer to a serving platter and present on toothpicks with Remoulade Sauce on the side.

SERVES 4

Per serving: 95 calories; 16.0 grams protein; 3.5 grams carbohydrates; 1.8 grams fat (.9 gram fat from fish); 42 milligrams cholesterol; 450 milligrams sodium (without salting).

# CRABMEAT-STUFFED ARTICHOKE

The garlicky *aioli* adds zing to the crabmeat mixture without overpowering the crustacean's distinctive character.

  4 artichokes, cooked and cooled
  ½ pound cooked crabmeat, cartilage removed
  ½ cup Almost Aioli (page 7)
  1 head Bibb or Boston lettuce, separated into leaves

1. Gently pull open the center leaves of each artichoke. Pull out a few of the leaves, and with a small spoon or serrated knife remove and discard the choke; set artichokes aside.

2. Combine crabmeat and Almost Aioli in a small bowl and mix thoroughly.

3. Spoon crabmeat mixture into the center of each artichoke.

4. Place lettuce leaves on plates and top with artichokes. Serve at room temperature or slightly chilled.

SERVES 4

Per serving: 125 calories; 16.0 grams protein; 15.5 grams carbohydrates; 1.2 grams fat (.7 gram fat from fish); 32 milligrams cholesterol; 435 milligrams sodium (without salting).

# CHILLED SHRIMP
# WITH GINGERED CARROTS

Shredded carrots with ginger splashed with rice wine vinegar and fragrant sesame oil somehow coaxes the true essence of shrimp. Marvelous for the steamy days of summer, it's a perfect prelude to any festive dinner.

1 teaspoon fresh lemon juice
$1/4$ teaspoon hot pepper flakes
$1/2$ pound large shrimp, rinsed
6 thin carrots, cut into pieces
1 small piece ginger root (about 1 inch), peeled and cut in pieces
1 tablespoon rice wine vinegar
2 teaspoons sesame oil

1. Heat about 2 quarts of water in a large pot. Add lemon juice and hot pepper flakes and bring to a boil. Add shrimp to water, allow water to return to a boil, and cook for about 3 minutes or until shrimp are cooked through.

2. Drain and transfer shrimp to a colander and place under cold running water. Let cool to room temperature, then peel and devein shrimp and refrigerate to chill.

3. Using a food processor, grate carrots and ginger. Spoon into a small bowl.

4. Combine rice wine vinegar and sesame oil. Mix

well and stir into carrot-ginger mixture. Allow mixture to stand for 30 minutes to blend flavors.

5. Spoon carrot-ginger mixture into the center of a serving platter and mound. Arrange shrimp around mound and serve.

SERVES 4

Per serving: 115 calories; 12.2 grams protein; 8.5 grams carbohydrates; 3.5 grams fat (1.0 gram fat from fish); 87 milligrams cholesterol; 110 milligrams sodium (without salting).

# STIR-FRIED SCALLOPS
# AND VEGETABLES

Aside from fitting perfectly into the healthy, low fat way of life, scallops take to just about every type of cooking method. In this Chinese-influenced recipe, they are quickly stir-fried with fresh, crunchy vegetables, including celery, water chestnuts, snow peas, and scallions. The addition of the immensely flavorful five-spice powder (a combination of cinnamon, cloves, fennel seed, star anise, and Szechuan peppercorns, long a staple in Asian cuisine) infuses this dish with a wonderful pungency.

    1 tablespoon vegetable oil
    1 small onion, cut into rings
    2 stalks celery, coarsely chopped
    4 scallions, cut into $1/2$-inch lengths
    6 fresh or canned water chestnuts, sliced, or $1/2$ cup
        sliced jicama
    $1/2$ cup fresh snow peas or sugar snap peas
    $3/4$ pound bay scallops, or quartered sea scallops
    1 teaspoon cornstarch
    $1/4$ cup Low Fat Chicken Stock (page 3), canned low
        sodium broth, or cold water
    $1/4$ teaspoon 5-spice powder or to taste

    1. Heat vegetable oil in a large nonstick skillet. Add vegetables and cook over medium-high heat, stirring, for 2 minutes.

2. Add scallops to skillet and cook, stirring, for an additional 4 minutes or until scallops are nearly cooked through.

3. Combine cornstarch, stock, and 5 spices in a small bowl. Mix well and stir into skillet. Continue cooking for about 2 minutes or until sauce has thickened and scallops are cooked through. Serve hot.

SERVES 4

Per serving: 140 calories; 15.5 grams protein; 10.0 grams carbohydrates; 4.2 grams fat (.6 gram fat from fish); 27 milligrams cholesterol; 165 milligrams sodium (without salting).

# LETTUCE-WRAPPED
# SHRIMP ROLLS

Egg rolls are a great favorite and make a wonderful appetizer, but the usual recipe calls for deep frying, adding unneeded fat to a meal. Here the spicy filling is wrapped in lettuce leaves rather than in the usual egg roll skins and the result is a lot of flavor with far less fat. And everyone seems to enjoy rolling their own.

2 teaspoons sesame oil
2 teaspoons low sodium soy sauce
1 tablespoon grated ginger
1 stalk celery, finely diced
1 carrot, finely diced
1 small red bell pepper, thinly sliced
4 scallions, thinly sliced
$\frac{1}{2}$ cup shredded cabbage
1 clove garlic, pressed
$\frac{1}{2}$ pound medium shrimp, shelled, deveined, and diced
$\frac{1}{4}$ cup rice wine vinegar
$\frac{1}{2}$ teaspoon hot pepper sauce or to taste
1 tablespoon minced fresh cilantro
1 head green leaf or iceberg lettuce, rinsed, dried, and
    separated into leaves

1. Combine oil, soy sauce, and ginger in a large nonstick skillet over medium heat. Add all the vegetables and garlic and stir to combine. Cover and cook

about 3 minutes or until vegetables are just wilted. Using a slotted spoon, transfer vegetables to a large bowl.

2. Add shrimp, rice wine vinegar, hot sauce, and cilantro to skillet. Cook, uncovered, stirring, for about 3 minutes or until shrimp are cooked through.

3. Combine shrimp and vegetables and mix well. Refrigerate for 30 minutes.

4. To serve, present a pile of lettuce leaves and a mound of shrimp-vegetable mixture. Let everyone prepare their own shrimp roll.

SERVES 4

Per serving: 130 calories; 14.0 grams protein; 9.5 grams carbohydrates; 3.8 grams fat (1.0 gram fat from fish); 87 milligrams cholesterol; 215 milligrams sodium (without salting).

# BAKED OYSTERS WITH WATERCRESS

My recipe for baked oysters goes easy on the bread crumbs, which I often have found to be served soggy, and heavier on the proportion of watercress.

  24 oysters
    1 tablespoon fine bread crumbs
  1/4 cup minced watercress
    1 tablespoon olive oil
      Freshly ground black pepper to taste
      Fresh lemon juice to taste

1. Preheat oven to 500° F.
2. Scrub oysters and shuck. Place each oyster on a half shell and arrange in a shallow baking pan.
3. Combine bread crumbs and watercress. Mix well and spoon over oysters. Drizzle with olive oil and season with pepper to taste. Bake for 4 minutes. Moisten with lemon juice to taste before serving.

SERVES 4
Per serving: 90 calories; 6.0 grams protein; 3.7 grams carbohydrates; 5.6 grams fat (2.1 grams fat from fish); 46 milligrams cholesterol; 100 milligrams sodium (without salting).

# CALAMARI IN SAVORY TOMATO SAUCE WITH CAPERS AND OLIVES

A terrific starter on its own, this dish makes an excellent main dish for four served over the pasta of your choice. The squid (calamari) toughens quickly so avoid overcooking.

    1 tablespoon olive oil
    1 medium onion, diced
    2 large cloves garlic, finely minced
    1 large can (28 ounces) no-salt-added crushed
        tomatoes
    1/2 cup chopped fresh Italian parsley
    1 teaspoon dried oregano
    1/2 teaspoon hot red pepper flakes or to taste
    2 tablespoons capers, rinsed and drained
    4 pitted black olives, diced
        Salt and freshly ground pepper to taste
    1/2 pound cleaned and trimmed calamari (squid), cut
        into circles or strips

1. Heat oil in a large nonstick skillet. Add onion and garlic and stir over medium heat for about 2 minutes or until softened but not browned.

2. Add all remaining ingredients, except squid, to skillet and let simmer, stirring frequently, for about 8 minutes or until liquid is slightly reduced and

thickened. Taste and add salt and pepper if needed, or adjust seasonings to taste.

3. Add squid and cook for 3 to 5 minutes or until just cooked through. Remove from heat and serve immediately on individual dishes.

SERVES 6
Per serving: 100 calories; 7.5 grams protein; 10.0 grams carbohydrates; 3.4 grams fat (.5 gram fat from fish); 88 milligrams cholesterol; 115 milligrams sodium (without salting).

# SHERRIED SHRIMP ESPAÑOL

This recipe features dry sherry, the famed fortified wine of Spain, as the base for an herbed marinade for the shrimp that are then briefly broiled, once again benefiting from the complexly flavored marinade.

Excellent as a first course, this shrimp dish could easily serve as an elegant luncheon for two accompanied by salad and a hot bread.

*1/2 cup dry sherry (not cooking wine)*
*2 teaspoons olive oil*
*6 large cloves garlic, pressed*
*1/4 teaspoon dried chervil*
*1/4 teaspoon dried tarragon*
*1/4 cup chopped fresh parsley*
*1/4 cup chopped fresh chives*
*1/2 pound medium shrimp, shelled and deveined*
*Salt and freshly ground pepper to taste*

1. Combine all ingredients, except shrimp and salt and pepper, in a small bowl and mix until thoroughly combined.

2. Place shrimp in a shallow dish and add sherry mixture. Allow shrimp to marinate, refrigerated, for 4 hours, turning shrimp frequently in marinade.

3. Preheat broiler to high.

4. Divide shrimp and marinade among 4 ovenproof ramekins, or place all in an ovenproof dish.

Broil about 4 inches from heat, turning shrimp once. Cook about 5 minutes or until slightly browned. Season with salt and pepper and serve.

SERVES 4

Per serving: 95 calories; 12.5 grams protein; 3.5 grams carbohydrates; 3.5 grams fat (1.0 gram fat from fish); 87 milligrams cholesterol; 90 milligrams sodium (without salting).

# CURRIED HALIBUT SALAD

A dandy change from tuna fish salad, this dish can be made in under a half hour, even when you start from "scratch." The recipe calls for halibut, but any fish fillet or leftover steamed or poached fish will work quite well.

1½ pounds halibut fillets
2 large shallots
2 stalks celery, halved
½ cup Almost Aioli (page 7)
2 teaspoons mild or hot curry powder or to taste
Salt and freshly ground pepper to taste
1 medium head Belgian endive
½ cup fresh pineapple chunks

1. Pour water into the bottom of a steamer. Place fish on steaming rack and cover. Bring water to a boil and steam for about 6 minutes or until fish flakes when tested with a fork. Remove fish from steamer and allow to cool.

2. Cut fish into large chunks and place in a food processor. Add shallots, celery, Almost Aioli, and curry powder. Process until ingredients are blended and finely chopped. Taste to adjust seasonings or add salt and pepper if desired.

3. Separate endive into individual leaves and place leaves around the outside rim of a serving platter. Spoon pineapple on and around leaves.

4. Mound fish mixture in the center of the platter and refrigerate for 15 minutes before serving.

SERVES 6

Per serving: 160 calories; 25.5 grams protein; 7.5 grams carbohydrates; 2.9 grams fat (2.4 grams fat from fish); 37 milligrams cholesterol; 110 milligrams sodium (without salting).

# PASTA
# AND RICE

# PENNE WITH SHRIMP, SPINACH, AND SWEET PEPPERS

If desired, another medium-size, sturdy pasta, such as ziti, may be substituted.

    1 tablespoon olive oil
    1 large onion, diced
    2 medium red bell peppers, trimmed, seeded, and cut
        into thin 1-inch strips
    ½ pound medium penne
    1 clove garlic, minced
    ½ cup Low Fat Chicken Stock (page 3) or canned low
        sodium broth
    10 ounces spinach, rinsed, trimmed, and coarsely
        chopped
    ½ pound shrimp, rinsed, shelled, and deveined
        Salt and freshly ground pepper to taste

1. Heat oil in a large nonstick skillet. Add onion and red pepper and cook, stirring frequently, over medium heat for 8 minutes or until onion is golden.

2. While vegetables cook, put pasta in a large pot full of boiling water. Cover.

3. When onion is golden, add garlic to skillet and cook for 1 minute. Add stock or broth and bring to a simmer. Add spinach and cook, stirring frequently, for about 2 minutes or until spinach starts to wilt.

4. Add shrimp to skillet and cook over medium

heat, stirring, for 5 minutes or until shrimp is just cooked. Reduce heat to low.

5. When pasta is cooked, drain and add to skillet with shrimp and vegetables. Season to taste with salt and pepper, toss gently to blend ingredients, and serve immediately.

SERVES 4

Per serving: 345 calories; 21.0 grams protein; 52.5 grams carbohydrates; 5.7 grams fat (1.0 gram fat from fish); 86 milligrams cholesterol; 140 milligrams sodium (without salting).

# SAUTÉED WHITING WITH GREEN AND WHITE FETTUCCINE

Along with monkfish, skate, sea robins, and dog-fish, whiting once basked in relative obscurity. Currently, these formerly disdained, so-called "trash fish" are riding a tidal wave of popularity.

Here, the firm-textured, delicately flavored whiting rests on sagaciously sauced white and green fettuccine. Serve with a salad of green and wax beans.

1 pound fillet of whiting, cut into 2-inch strips
1/4 cup all-purpose flour
1/4 teaspoon freshly ground pepper
1 tablespoon vegetable or olive oil
1 cup Low Fat Chicken Stock (page 3) or canned low
    sodium broth
1/2 teaspoon dried sage
1/4 pound green fettuccine, cooked al dente
1/4 pound white fettuccine, cooked al dente
1/2 cup shredded red leaf lettuce
    Salt to taste

1. Dredge fish in flour, shaking off excess. Season with pepper.

2. Heat oil in a large nonstick skillet. Add whiting and sauté over high heat, turning from side to side

until browned, about 3 to 4 minutes. Remove with a slotted spatula and drain on paper towels.

3. Add stock and sage to skillet. Cover, and bring to a simmer over low heat. Add green and white fettuccine to skillet and toss to combine. Remove from heat and stir in lettuce. Taste and adjust seasonings and add salt if necessary.

4. Spoon fettuccine combination onto a heated serving platter. Place sautéed whiting on top of fettuccine and serve.

SERVES 4

Per serving: 350 calories; 26.0 grams protein; 49.0 grams carbohydrates; 5.6 grams fat (1.1 grams fat from fish); 57 milligrams cholesterol; 85 milligrams sodium (without salting).

# LEMON SOLE
## WITH FARFELLE
## AND GREEN PEAS

Farfelle with green peas is a northern Italian favorite, traditionally combined with a butter and cream sauce and perhaps some prosciutto. Here, I've eliminated the rich sauce opting instead to complement the pasta and peas with elegant sole and a lovely low fat emulsion of wine, stock, and the noble leek. A bowl of cauliflower/broccoli florets would be a terrific sole-mate.

2 teaspoons vegetable oil
$1/4$ cup dry white wine
2 cups Low Fat Chicken Stock (page 3) or canned low
    sodium broth
1 cup fresh or frozen and thawed green peas
1 leek, white and tender greens, well-rinsed and finely
    chopped
1 pound lemon sole fillets, cut into large pieces
$1/2$ pound small farfelle (pasta bows), cooked al dente
    Salt and freshly ground pepper to taste

1. Heat oil in a large skillet. Add wine and cook for 2 minutes. Add stock and bring to a simmer. Add peas and leeks and cook until peas are tender.

2. Add lemon sole to skillet, cover, and cook for about 5 minutes or until fish is done.

3. Place cooked pasta bows on a heated serving

platter. Spoon contents of skillet over pasta and toss. Season with salt and pepper to taste and serve.

SERVES 4

Per serving: 395 calories; 31.7 grams protein; 55.0 grams carbohydrates; 5.3 grams fat (1.4 grams fat from fish); 55 milligrams cholesterol; 140 milligrams sodium (without salting).

# BRAISED TUNA WITH CAVATELLI

The addition of sweet peppers, onion, garlic, and a robust sauce to cubes of tuna fish creates a bold and low fat combination with cavatelli or, if that is not available, orecchiette, farfelle, shells, or ziti.

   1 medium onion
   2 cloves garlic
   1 small green or red bell pepper, cored, seeded, and
       cut into chunks
     Olive oil cooking spray
   2 cans (6-ounce) no-salt-added tomato paste
   5 cans (6-ounce) water
   1 tablespoon minced fresh basil or 1 teaspoon dried
   1/2 teaspoon dried oregano
   1/2 teaspoon hot red pepper flakes or to taste
   3/4 pound tuna fillets, cubed
     Salt to taste
   3/4 pound cavatelli, cooked al dente
   1 tablespoon minced fresh basil or parsley

   1. Place onion, garlic, and bell pepper in a food processor and chop coarsely.

   2. Heat a large nonstick skillet coated with cooking spray. Add chopped vegetables and cook over medium heat, stirring, for 2 minutes. Add tomato paste, water, basil, oregano, and hot pepper to skillet. Stir well to blend ingredients. Reduce heat to low and simmer, stirring frequently, for 20 minutes.

3. Add tuna and simmer for an additional 10 minutes, stirring occasionally. Taste and adjust seasonings and add salt if desired.

4. Place cooked cavatelli in a large heated serving bowl. Spoon tuna and sauce over pasta and gently toss. Sprinkle with basil or parsley and serve.

SERVES 6

Per serving: 360 calories; 22.5 grams protein; 57.0 grams carbohydrates; 4.5 grams fat (2.8 grams fat from fish); 22 milligrams cholesterol; 65 milligrams sodium (without salting).

# SPINACH LINGUINE
# WITH SCALLOPS AND
# TOMATOES

Don't let the simplicity of this dish fool you. The ingredients are there to complement the delicate flavor of the scallops. A sophisticated and low fat "fast food," scallops are sold shucked, trimmed, and ready for the pan, and take only minutes to cook.

An eggless Caesar-type salad would be a perfect foil for this lovely dish.

10 ripe fresh plum tomatoes, diced
 2 cloves garlic, pressed
 2 tablespoons chopped fresh basil
   Salt and freshly ground pepper to taste
 4 teaspoons olive oil
 1/2 pound bay scallops or sea scallops cut in half,
       rinsed and patted dry
 1/2 pound spinach linguine, cooked al dente

1. Combine tomatoes, garlic, basil, salt, pepper, and 2 teaspoons oil in a bowl. Mix and allow ingredients to blend for 1 hour or longer.

2. Heat remaining 2 teaspoons oil in a medium nonstick skillet. Add scallops and sauté for 3 to 4 minutes, turning to brown slightly on all sides. Be careful not to overcook scallops.

3. Place cooked linguine in a heated serving bowl.

Spoon tomato mixture over pasta and toss to combine.

4. Remove scallops from skillet with a slotted spoon, arrange on top of pasta, and serve.

Serves 4

Per serving: 335 calories; 18.0 grams protein; 52.5 grams carbohydrates; 6.3 grams fat (.4 gram fat from fish); 18 milligrams cholesterol; 115 milligrams sodium (without salting).

# DILLED SHRIMP
# WITH ANGEL HAIR

Scandinavians have long treasured the coupling of
the fernlike herb called dill and fish, particularly
salmon and shrimp. And although my recipe calls
for the aromatic dill and shrimp combination, the
Norse had little to do with its creation—what with
angel hair (cappellini) pasta as a third partner.

*1 cup Low Fat Chicken Stock (page 3) or canned low
    sodium broth*
*¼ cup dry white wine*
*¼ cup white wine vinegar*
*½ pound shrimp, peeled, deveined, and cut in half*
*½ cup plus 1 tablespoon chopped fresh dill weed
    Salt and freshly ground pepper to taste*
*½ pound angel hair pasta, cooked al dente*
*1 teaspoon olive oil*

1. Combine stock or broth, wine, and vinegar in a
large saucepan. Bring to a boil, add shrimp, and simmer for 3 minutes.

2. Remove saucepan from heat and stir in ½ cup
of dill. Return to heat for 1 to 2 minutes, or until
shrimp are cooked through. Season to taste with salt
and pepper.

3. Place pasta in a heated serving bowl. Pour
shrimp and sauce over pasta and toss gently to mix.

Drizzle olive oil over pasta, sprinkle with remaining tablespoon of dill, and serve.

SERVES 4

Per serving: 300 calories; 19.5 grams protein; 48.0 grams carbohydrates; 3.5 grams fat (1.0 gram fat from fish); 86 milligrams cholesterol; 120 milligrams sodium (without salting).

# CLAMS WITH PENNE
# IN LEMON SAUCE

Notice this recipe is called "Clams with Penne in Lemon Sauce." It is *not* your everyday, run-of-the-mill pasta with clam sauce! Here, the clams are showcased—with the pasta and topping acting as their able augmenters. Steamed until they open, the clams are added whole at the very last minute to the penne mixture, thus retaining their texture and taste.

2 dozen littleneck or cherrystone clams, scrubbed, rinsed, and drained
3/4 cup dry white wine
1 teaspoon olive oil
3 shallots, minced
2 cloves garlic, pressed
1/4 teaspoon hot red pepper flakes or to taste
1/4 cup Low Fat Chicken Stock (page 3) or canned low sodium broth
1 1/2 tablespoons fresh lemon juice
1/2 pound penne or other sturdy pasta, cooked al dente
1 tablespoon chopped fresh parsley

1. Place clams in a large pot. Add wine, cover, and steam over high heat for 8 to 10 minutes or until shells have opened. Remove clams from liquid and discard any clams that have not opened. Allow to

cool, then remove clams from shell. Strain liquid and reserve.

2. Heat oil in a large nonstick skillet. Add shallots, garlic, and red pepper flakes and cook, stirring, for 1 minute. Add reserved clam liquid, stock or broth, and lemon juice. Stir and heat through.

3. Add cooked penne to skillet and toss to combine. Add clams and toss again. Transfer to a heated bowl, garnish with parsley, and serve.

SERVES 4

Per serving: 285 calories; 15.0 grams protein; 49.5 grams carbohydrates; 2.8 grams fat (.6 gram fat from fish); 18 milligrams cholesterol; 45 milligrams sodium (without salting).

# SCALLOPS WITH RICE, BASQUE STYLE

Perhaps because the Basque region straddles the French and Spanish Pyrenees, its people produce a cuisine that reflects that rugged terrain. Famous for imaginative stews and casseroles, I've adapted one of their marvelous seafood and rice dishes, which is usually prepared with chorizos and pimientos. My version omits the sausage and uses mixed fresh sweet peppers.

Scallops are intended only as a suggestion here. Any white, firm-textured fish or shrimp would also work well. Hearts of lettuce would be a pleasant sidebar.

    1 tablespoon olive oil
    4 large shallots, minced
      Salt and freshly ground pepper to taste
1¼ cups white or brown rice
    4 cups Low Fat Chicken Stock (page 3) or canned low
      sodium broth
    3 small mixed bell peppers (green, red, yellow, or
      combination), trimmed and diced
    1 pound scallops, rinsed and cut into ½-inch pieces

1. Heat oil in a large deep skillet or stockpot. Add shallots and cook over medium heat, stirring frequently, for 5 minutes or until softened but not browned. Season to taste with salt and pepper.

2. Stir in rice and add stock. Bring to a boil, then reduce heat to low, cover, and simmer for 15 minutes.

3. Gently stir in bell peppers and simmer, covered, for an additional 10 minutes or until rice is just tender.

4. Fold in scallops and simmer, uncovered, for about 5 minutes or until scallops are cooked through and rice is tender. Transfer to a heated platter and serve.

SERVES 4

Per serving: 400 calories; 25.0 grams protein; 62.5 grams carbohydrates; 5.3 grams fat (.8 gram fat from fish); 36 milligrams cholesterol; 250 milligrams sodium (without salting).

# CRABMEAT RISOTTO
# WITH ASPARAGUS AND OLIVES

Yes, risotto requires a degree of patience and vigilance, but the results are well worth the effort. Present this elegant dish proudly to your most favored guests and wait for the compliments.

4 cups Low Fat Chicken Stock (page 3) or canned low
    sodium broth, approximate
1 tablespoon fresh lemon juice
1 tablespoon olive oil
6 shallots, minced
1 clove garlic, minced
1¼ cups arborio rice
¾ pound fresh or frozen crabmeat, cartilage removed,
    cut into bite-size chunks
8 stalks asparagus, tough stems removed, cut in half
    lengthwise, then diagonally into 1-inch pieces
6 pitted black olives, thinly sliced
    Salt and freshly ground pepper to taste
1 tablespoon minced fresh Italian parsley

1. In a large saucepan bring stock and lemon juice to a slow simmer.
2. Heat oil in a large, deep nonstick skillet. Add shallots and garlic and stir over medium heat for about 2 minutes or until softened. Add rice and cook for an additional minute, stirring to coat the grains.
3. Add a ladleful (about ½ cup) of the simmering

stock to the rice in skillet and stir over medium heat until stock has been absorbed. Continue to add stock by the ladleful and to stir, for about 30 minutes or until rice is done (it should be creamy outside but still a touch firm to the bite inside; you may not use all the stock). If necessary, raise heat to keep mixture at a simmer, but do not let boil.

4. About 8 minutes before rice is done, add crabmeat, asparagus, olives, and salt and pepper to rice and stir gently, continuing to add stock until ingredients are cooked.

5. Remove from heat, stir in parsley, transfer to heated bowl or platter and serve.

SERVES 4

Per serving: 385 calories; 22.5 grams protein; 60.0 grams carbohydrates; 5.8 grams fat (1.0 gram fat from fish); 47 milligrams cholesterol; 570 milligrams sodium (without salting).

# LOBSTER WITH RICE AND ROASTED PEPPER

When I eat this dish, I feel I've just died and gone to heaven! Lobster and roasted pepper slices tossed into a richly—but not "rich"—flavored rice and topped with beautiful wedges of tomato is not only super-delicious, it is super-looking.

2 medium red bell peppers
1 tablespoon vegetable oil
4 shallots, minced
2 cloves garlic, pressed
1/4 cup chopped fresh basil or Italian parsley
    Pinch cayenne pepper or to taste
1 cup rice
2 1/2 cups Fish Stock (page 5) or Low Fat Chicken Stock
    (page 3) or canned low sodium broth
3/4 pound cooked lobster meat (from 2 lobsters, about
    1 1/2 pounds each)
    Salt and freshly ground pepper to taste
1 large ripe tomato, cut into eighths

1. Roast red peppers by charring skin on all sides under broiler or over gas flame. Place blackened peppers in a paper bag, close bag and let stand until cool enough to handle. Peel off charred skin (this is easiest done with wet hands). Core and seed peppers. Cut roasted peppers into thin slices and reserve.

2. Heat oil in a large, deep nonstick skillet. Add shallots, garlic, basil, and cayenne and cook over medium heat, stirring, for 1 minute. Add rice and stir for about 1 minute or until rice is translucent.

3. Add stock to skillet. Reduce heat to low, cover, and cook for about 20 minutes or until rice is tender. Add roasted pepper slices and lobster meat and toss gently. Taste, adjust seasonings and add salt and pepper if desired. Cover and cook briefly, until ingredients are heated through. Spoon onto a heated platter, arrange tomato wedges on top, and serve.

Serves 4

Per serving: 335 calories; 22.5 grams protein; 50.5 grams carbohydrates; 4.7 grams fat (.5 gram fat from fish); 62 milligrams cholesterol; 375 milligrams sodium (without salting).

# SEAFOOD PAELLA

Traditionally, paella (py-AY-yah) is a Spanish dish made with saffron-flavored rice combined with a variety of meats and shellfish, garlic, onion, and peas. It is named for the wide, two-handled pan— which is also called paella—in which it's prepared and served.

This is a fish-only paella, which reduces the fat and calories of the classic. My recipe calls for a teaspoon of crushed saffron threads (that most pricey of all seasonings) and, fortunately, a little goes a long way. Unfortunately, there is no good substitute for the real McCoy.

Truly a one-dish meal, paella needs no accompaniment, save for an icy pitcher of sangria or iced tea to pass around.

2 cups Low Fat Chicken Stock (page 3) or canned low sodium broth
2 cups water
1 cup dry white wine
$1/2$ pound fish fillets (sole, flounder, cod, whiting)
$1/2$ pound large shrimp, rinsed
$1/2$ pound scallops, rinsed
2 dozen fresh small clams, scrubbed and rinsed
1 tablespoon olive oil
1 small red onion, diced
2 cloves garlic, minced
2 stalks celery, diced

1 teaspoon crushed saffron threads
1/2 teaspoon hot pepper flakes or to taste, optional
1 1/2 cups white long-grain rice
3 tablespoons minced fresh parsley
   Salt and freshly ground pepper to taste
4 medium tomatoes, chopped
1 green bell pepper, trimmed and diced
2 ounces pimientos, drained and diced
1 1/2 cups fresh or frozen and thawed green peas
   Juice from 1 large lemon

1. Combine stock, water, and wine in a soup pot and bring to a boil. Add fish fillets, shrimp, scallops, and clams. Using a slotted spoon, remove fish and seafood as it is cooked, discarding any unopened clams, and set aside. Keep cooking liquid simmering.

2. Heat oil in a paella pot or a large, deep nonstick skillet. Add onion, garlic, and celery, and stir over medium heat for 3 minutes. Stir in saffron, hot pepper flakes, if desired, and rice. Add hot cooking liquid, parsley, and salt and pepper to rice in skillet and stir gently. Cover and simmer over very low heat for 15 minutes.

3. While rice simmers, shell and devein shrimp and set aside.

4. Add tomatoes and green pepper to skillet and simmer an additional 10 to 15 minutes or until rice is tender.

5. Add pimientos, peas, and reserved seafood to skillet. Stir very gently, and continue to simmer for an additional 2 to 3 minutes or until all ingredients

are thoroughly heated. Sprinkle with lemon juice, taste and adjust seasonings if necessary, and serve.

SERVES 6

Per serving: 385 calories; 31.5 grams protein; 53.5 grams carbohydrates; 4.7 grams fat (1.6 grams fat from fish); 98 milligrams cholesterol; 210 milligrams sodium (without salting).

# THE MAIN COURSE:
## BAKED
## DISHES

# STUFFED MAHIMAHI

Also called "dolphinfish" and "donado," mahimahi is found in warm waters throughout the world. A moderately fat fish with tender, sweet flesh, the fillets in this recipe are stuffed with coarsely grated zucchini and carrot seasoned with a bit of orange juice, turmeric, and ginger.

I like to serve crisp-steamed snow peas and rice with this dish.

1 small zucchini, halved
1 small carrot, quartered
1 tablespoon orange juice
1/4 teaspoon ground turmeric
1/4 teaspoon ground ginger
1 pound mahimahi fillets
1/2 cup Low Fat Chicken Stock (page 3) or canned low
    sodium broth
    Salt and freshly ground pepper to taste
1/2 cup Light Rouille (page 6), optional

1. Preheat oven to 350° F.
2. Place zucchini, carrot, orange juice, turmeric, and ginger in a food processor and coarsely grate vegetables.
3. Spread one-quarter of vegetable mixture in center of a mahimahi fillet and roll, securing with a toothpick. Repeat with remaining vegetable mixture and fish.

4. Place fish fillets, seam-side down, in a nonstick baking pan. Pour stock over fish and season with salt and pepper. Bake, uncovered, for about 20 minutes or until fish is cooked through.

5. Transfer to a heated platter and serve with Light Rouille sauce on the side if desired.

SERVES 4

Per serving: 110 calories; 21.5 grams protein; 3.8 grams carbohydrates; 1.0 gram fat (.8 gram fat from fish); 83 milligrams cholesterol; 115 milligrams sodium (without salting).

# DRUNKEN POMPANO
# A LA PUERTA VALLARTA

The jalapeño or ancho pepper is what gives this Mexican-style preparation its kick (use rubber gloves when handling), while the vegetables and seasonings provide texture and good nutrition. But it is the six rounds of red wine that really makes this dish a knockout. (If alcohol is not your thing, there are dealcoholized dry red wines on the market that make credible substitutes.) If you can't find pompano, try mahimahi, swordfish, or snapper. The cooking times are approximately the same.

Go all the way and serve with some more South-of-the-Border treats such as black beans and rice, and steamed tortillas.

*2 teaspoons vegetable oil*
*1 small onion, finely chopped*
*1 clove garlic, pressed*
*2 large tomatoes, peeled and chopped*
*1 small jalapeño or ancho pepper, cored, seeded, and minced*
*¼ teaspoon ground cumin*
*¼ teaspoon dried oregano*
*1 teaspoon sugar*
*2 cups dry red wine*
*4 pompano fillets, each about 4 ounces*

1. Preheat oven to 350° F.

2. Heat oil in a medium nonstick skillet. Add onion and garlic and cook over medium-high heat, stirring, for 1 minute. Add tomatoes, jalapeño or ancho pepper, cumin, oregano and sugar, and bring to a simmer. Stir in wine and cook for 2 minutes.

3. Place pompano in a baking dish or casserole. Pour wine sauce over fish, cover, and bake for 10 to 15 minutes, or until fish is cooked through. Carefully remove fish to a platter and keep warm.

4. Transfer liquid to a saucepan and reduce to about 1 cup. Spoon sauce over fish and serve.

SERVES 4

Per serving: 250 calories; 22.0 grams protein; 10.5 grams carbohydrates; 12.8 grams fat (10.6 grams fat from fish); 57 milligrams cholesterol; 155 milligrams sodium (without salting).

# BLUEFISH BAKED
# IN GREEN TOMATO SAUCE

The green tomato sauce adds a piquant and different flavor to old reliable bluefish. I serve this dish with boiled potatoes and a quick-cooked seasonal vegetable.

    4 medium green tomatoes (about 1 pound), quartered
    1 small onion, halved
    1 clove garlic
    1/2 cup packed fresh cilantro or Italian parsley
       Salt and freshly ground pepper to taste
    4 fillets of bluefish, about 4 ounces each
       Juice of 1 large lemon

1. Preheat oven to 350° F.

2. Combine tomatoes, onion, garlic, and cilantro or parsley in a food processor and process until finely chopped. Season to taste.

3. Spoon half of tomato mixture on the bottom of a baking pan. Top with fish fillets, and cover fish with remainder of tomato sauce. Sprinkle with lemon juice. Bake until fish flakes easily with a fork, about 15 to 20 minutes.

4. Transfer fish and sauce to a heated serving platter or individual plates and serve immediately.

Serves 4

Per serving: 175 calories; 24.5 grams protein; 7.5 grams carbohydrates; 5.0 grams fat (4.8 grams fat from fish); 67 milligrams cholesterol; 85 milligrams sodium (without salting).

# BAKED WHOLE SEA BASS WITH ASIAN OYSTER SAUCE

As far as I'm concerned, oyster sauce could make paper towels appetizing to eat! Available in most supermarkets and Asian grocery stores, the dark-brown sauce imparts a special richness to dishes. Here, I use it with ginger, soy sauce, and tasty sesame oil in a marinade that also acts as the fish's cooking liquid. Radishes—which impart an interesting texture, taste, and color contrast—are added to the mixture after cooking.

Serve with a salad of fresh bean sprouts and french-cut green beans.

1 sea bass (about 2 to 2½ pounds), cleaned and left
   whole
1½ tablespoons peeled ginger root slivers
1 tablespoon low sodium soy sauce
1 tablespoon Asian oyster sauce
1 teaspoon sesame oil
   Vegetable oil cooking spray
1 cup Low Fat Chicken Stock (page 3) or canned low
   sodium broth
4 scallions, cut into ½-inch lengths
6 red radishes, thinly sliced
1 teaspoon cornstarch
2 tablespoons water

1. Cut slits into both sides of fish, about 2 inches apart. Insert ginger slivers into slits.

2. Combine soy sauce, oyster sauce, and sesame oil in small bowl. Mix until thoroughly blended and pour over fish. Allow fish to marinate in the refrigerator for 30 minutes, turning fish once in marinade.

3. Preheat oven to 425° F.

4. Lightly coat a shallow baking pan with cooking spray. Place fish with marinade in baking pan. Add stock and scallions. Cover with aluminum foil and bake until fish is cooked through, about 25 to 35 minutes, depending on size of fish. Transfer fish to a serving platter and keep warm.

5. Spoon sauce from baking pan into a saucepan and add radish. Bring sauce to a simmer. Dissolve cornstarch in water in a small bowl and add to sauce. Simmer until sauce thickens slightly. Pour over fish and serve.

SERVES 4

Per serving: 140 calories; 21.5 grams protein; 3.0 grams carbohydrates; 4.5 grams fat (2.3 grams from fish); 47 milligrams cholesterol; 225 milligrams sodium (without salting).

# MONKFISH HARLEQUINADE

This fish is alternately called "goosefish," "anglerfish," or "devilfish" because of its unattractive appearance when whole. But monkfish fillets are something I prize because of their firm, sweet, crustacean-like texture and flavor. I call this monkfish creation "Monkfish Harlequinade" because when prepared with colorful bell peppers, the dish is reminiscent of a Harlequin's bright costume.

Serve a watercress or arugula salad along with tiny, steamed red-skinned new potatoes.

1¼ pounds monkfish fillets
  1 large green bell pepper, cored, seeded, and cut into
      4 slices
  1 large red bell pepper, cored, seeded, and cut into 4
      slices
  1 large yellow bell pepper, cored, seeded, and cut into
      4 slices
  2 teaspoons olive oil
  1 tablespoon balsamic vinegar
¼ cup Low Fat Chicken Stock (page 3) or canned low
      sodium broth
¼ teaspoon ground cumin or to taste
  Salt and freshly ground pepper to taste
  Olive oil cooking spray

1. Place fish in a shallow dish and arrange bell pepper slices around fish.

2. In a small bowl, combine all remaining ingredients, except for cooking spray. Mix well and pour over fish and peppers. Marinate in refrigerator for 30 minutes, turning fish and peppers once.

3. Preheat oven to 425° F.

4. Coat a baking pan with cooking spray. Transfer fish and peppers to pan, and pour marinade over all. Bake for 10 minutes. Turn fish and peppers and continue baking for an additional 10 minutes, or until fillets are cooked through.

5. Transfer fish, peppers, and sauce to a heated platter and serve.

SERVES 4

Per serving: 150 calories; 21.5 grams protein; 4.0 grams carbohydrates; 5.2 grams fat (2.0 grams fat from fish); 35 milligrams cholesterol; 30 milligrams sodium (without salting).

# BAKED TUNA STEAKS
## WITH SUN-DRIED TOMATOES
## AND BASIL

This delicious dish is easy to make and takes very little time to prepare—you'll find it ideal when you're "running late" and have to deal with dinner in a hurry.

*Olive oil cooking spray*
*1/4 cup diced unseasoned sun-dried tomatoes, softened in boiling water and drained*
*1/4 cup chopped fresh basil*
*1 clove garlic, pressed*
*1/2 cup Low Fat Chicken Stock (page 3) or Fish Stock (page 5) or canned low sodium broth*
*4 tuna steaks, about 5 ounces each*
*Salt and freshly ground pepper to taste*

1. Preheat oven to 425° F.
2. Coat a nonstick skillet with cooking spray. Add sun-dried tomatoes, basil, and garlic and cook over low heat, stirring, for 1 minute. Add stock and bring to a simmer.
3. Coat a baking pan with cooking spray. Arrange tuna steaks in pan and season to taste with salt and pepper. Spoon tomato-basil mixture over tuna, and bake for about 15 minutes, or until fish flakes easily.
4. Transfer fish to a heated platter, top with sauce from baking pan, and serve.

SERVES 4

Per serving: 225 calories; 34.0 grams protein; 4.0 grams carbohydrates; 7.9 grams fat (7.0 grams fat from fish); 55 milligrams cholesterol; 75 milligrams sodium (without salting).

# TUNA STEAKS
# IN ORANGE SAUCE

I find that a good way to cut the fat in food preparation is by using fruit juices and spices, as illustrated in this scrumptious preparation. Simple, flavorful, and to the point, here is a way to enhance the tuna without a buttery sauce.

Accompany this dish with fragrant basmati rice and broccoli rabe or other deep-green colored vegetable.

$^1/_2$ cup orange juice
1 tablespoon fresh lime juice
2 teaspoons grated orange rind
$^1/_2$ teaspoon ground cardamom
4 tuna steaks, about 5 ounces each
   Salt and freshly ground pepper to taste
2 teaspoons cornstarch
2 tablespoons cold water
1 medium orange, peeled, seeded, and sectioned

1. Preheat oven to 425° F.
2. Combine orange juice, lime juice, orange rind, and cardamom in a small bowl and mix well.
3. Place tuna steaks in a nonstick baking pan. Pour orange juice mixture over fish and season to taste with salt and pepper. Bake for about 10 minutes or until fish is cooked through. Baste fish after 5 minutes and do not turn.

4. Transfer fish to a serving platter and keep warm. Pour pan juices into a small saucepan and bring to a simmer. Dissolve cornstarch in water, add to saucepan, and simmer until sauce thickens slightly.

5. Arrange orange slices around fish, spoon sauce over all, and serve.

SERVES 4

Per serving: 240 calories; 34.0 grams protein; 9.0 grams carbohydrates; 7.2 grams fat (7.0 grams fat from fish); 55 milligrams cholesterol; 55 milligrams sodium (without salting).

# COD STEAKS
# WITH GARLIC CONSERVE

An interesting paradox is that the longer you "stew" garlic, the mellower and more complex its taste becomes. The sixteen cloves of garlic called for in this recipe are gently simmered in seasoned stock before being paired with the fish, so the strong flavor and aroma is tamed while the essence of the garlic flavor remains. Be careful not to let the garlic brown or it will take on a bitter taste.

Just about any pasta, potato, or rice dish would be good with the cod.

16 large cloves garlic
1 cup Low Fat Chicken Stock (page 3) or canned low
    sodium broth
1 bay leaf
1/4 teaspoon ground cumin
1/4 teaspoon dried oregano
1 2-inch piece orange peel
1 small tomato, peeled and diced
2 tablespoons chopped fresh basil
4 cod steaks or fillets, about 5 ounces each
    Salt and freshly ground pepper to taste
4 lemon wedges
2 tomatoes, quartered

1. Peel garlic and place whole cloves in a saucepan. Add stock, bay leaf, cumin, and oregano. Cover

and simmer over low heat for 20 minutes. If necessary, add more stock—do not let garlic brown. Remove from heat and allow to cool. You now have garlic conserve.

2. Meanwhile, preheat oven to 450° F.

3. Pour boiling water over orange peel, let stand 1 minute, then drain. Cut orange peel into 4 pieces. Combine peel with tomato and basil and mix well.

4. Prepare 4 pieces of baking parchment paper or foil, each about 12 × 8 inches. Thinly slice 2 cloves of garlic and spread in center of each. Place 1 fish steak on top of sliced garlic cloves and top with one-quarter of orange-tomato mixture. Season to taste with salt and pepper. Fold parchment or foil over fish, sealing tightly. Place fish packets in a shallow baking pan, and bake for about 15 minutes, or until fish is cooked to your taste.

5. Unwrap fish and transfer to heated dinner plates. Garnish each fish steak with 2 cloves garlic, 1 lemon wedge, and half of a quartered tomato.

SERVES 4

Per serving: 170 calories; 26.5 grams protein; 14.0 grams carbohydrates; 1.5 grams fat (1.0 gram fat from fish); 61 milligrams cholesterol; 110 milligrams sodium (without salting).

# SOLE ROULADES
# WITH CAPER-YOGURT SAUCE

They say great things come in small packages, and this delightful dish proves the adage. A combination of chopped vegetables and seasonings are spread on fillets of sole that are rolled, baked, and topped with a parsley, garlic and yogurt sauce to which capers are added.

Orzo or egg barley and a slaw of julienned cucumbers and carrots would go nicely with the fish.

Vegetable oil cooking spray
1 medium tomato, peeled, seeded, and chopped
2 tablespoons chopped onion
1 teaspoon ground cumin
1 tablespoon minced fresh cilantro (coriander) or
   $^{1}/_{2}$ teaspoon dried
1 pound grey sole fillets
$^{1}/_{2}$ cup packed fresh parsley
$^{1}/_{2}$ cup nonfat plain yogurt
2 cloves garlic
3 tablespoons capers, rinsed and drained
1 lemon, quartered

1. Preheat oven to 400° F. Coat a baking pan with cooking spray and set aside.

2. Combine tomato, onion, cumin, and cilantro in a small bowl and mix well. Spoon equal amounts of tomato mixture in the center of each fillet and roll.

Place fillets, seam-side down, in prepared pan. Cover with foil and bake for about 15 minutes, or until fish is cooked through.

3. While fish bakes, puree parsley, yogurt, and garlic in a food processor. Transfer to a saucepan, add capers, and heat until just warm.

4. Place baked fish on a heated platter or individual plates and spoon yogurt sauce over fish. Serve with lemon wedges.

SERVES 4

Per serving: 140 calories; 23.0 grams protein; 7.5 grams carbohydrates; 2.3 grams fat (1.4 grams fat from fish); 55 milligrams cholesterol; 200 milligrams sodium (without salting).

# FILLET OF MACKEREL ROSEMARY

The sauce in this recipe, with its perfume of rosemary, is also composed of onion, shallots, garlic, tomatoes, and dry white wine. When served over the distinctively flavored mackerel (a cold-water fish thought to be particularly high in Omega-3) it makes an elegant and healthy main course.

    1 pound Atlantic mackerel fillets
      Vegetable oil cooking spray
    1 small onion, chopped
    2 large shallots, chopped
    1 clove garlic, minced
    2 medium tomatoes, peeled and chopped
    1 teaspoon chopped fresh rosemary or $^1/_2$ teaspoon
      dried
    1 cup dry white wine
      Salt and freshly ground pepper to taste
$^1/_4$ cup finely chopped fresh parsley
    1 lemon, cut into 4 wedges

1. Preheat oven to 400° F. Coat a baking dish or ovenproof casserole with cooking spray and set aside.

2. Rinse fish and pat dry. Place fish fillets in prepared baking dish. Distribute onion, shallots, garlic, and tomatoes over and around fish. Add rosemary

and white wine and season to taste. Bake for about
15 minutes or until fish is cooked through.

3. Carefully transfer fish fillets to a serving platter
and let cool.

4. Spoon sauce from baking dish into a saucepan.
Bring to a boil, and cook over high heat until the
sauce thickens and is reduced. Allow sauce to cool.
Spoon over fish and serve at room temperature, garnished with parsley and lemon.

SERVES 4
Per serving: 290 calories; 22.5 grams protein; 12.5 grams
carbohydrates; 16.8 grams fat (15.8 grams fat from fish);
80 milligrams cholesterol; 115 milligrams sodium (without salting).

# OVEN-FRIED HADDOCK WITH GARLIC-YOGURT CRUMB CRUST

Haddock is a delicious, big-flaked white fish with a subtle sweetness. The garlicky yogurt mixture and bread-crumb coating bring out the flavor of the haddock in this hearty yet sophisticated dish.

Serve it with a large salad of mixed lettuces, such as red oak, Bibb, Boston, and butterhead.

*1 pound haddock fillets*
*3 tablespoons low fat plain yogurt*
*2 cloves garlic, pressed*
*1 tablespoon finely minced scallions*
*1 tablespoon finely minced fresh Italian parsley*
  *Salt and freshly ground pepper to taste*
*1 cup dry bread crumbs, made from 2 slices dried*
   *firm white bread*
  *Olive oil cooking spray*

1. Rinse haddock and pat dry. If fillets are large, cut into even pieces and set aside.

2. In a small bowl combine all remaining ingredients, except bread crumbs, and stir until well-blended. Spread yogurt mixture over all sides of fish and refrigerate for 30 minutes.

3. Preheat oven to 375° F.

4. Coat fish thoroughly with bread crumbs and place in a single layer on a shallow baking pan

coated with cooking spray. Bake for 10 to 15 minutes or until coating is golden and fish is cooked through. Serve hot.

SERVES 4

Per serving: 150 calories; 24.0 grams protein; 7.8 grams carbohydrates; 2.3 grams fat (.8 gram fat from fish); 66 milligrams cholesterol; 170 milligrams sodium (without salting).

# MONKFISH
# AND LEEK CASSEROLE

The surprise ingredient here is mint—which adds
an unexpected bit of zest to the casserole. You will
find this an excellent one-dish dinner for four.

    2 medium potatoes, peeled and diced
    1 medium carrot, diced
    ½ tablespoon olive oil
    4 leeks, white part and tender greens, well rinsed and
        chopped
    1 stalk celery, diced
    6 medium mushrooms, wiped clean and sliced
    ½ cup dry white wine
    1 tablespoon fresh lemon juice
    ¾ cup Low Fat Chicken Stock (page 3) or low sodium
        broth or water
      Salt and freshly ground pepper to taste
    ½ teaspoon dried mint
    1 pound monkfish, cut into 1-inch pieces
    1 cup bread crumbs, made from 2 slices dried firm
        white bread

1. Preheat oven to 375° F.

2. In a small saucepan, add potatoes and carrot to
boiling water and cook for 10 to 15 minutes or until
just tender; remove from heat, drain, and set aside.

3. While vegetables cook, heat oil in a large nonstick skillet. Add leeks and celery and cook over me-

dium heat, stirring frequently, for 2 minutes. Add mushrooms and cook for an additional 3 minutes.

4. Stir wine, lemon juice, stock, salt, pepper, and mint into skillet. Bring to a boil, then reduce heat to low and simmer gently, stirring frequently, for 5 minutes. Gently stir in monkfish, reserved potatoes and carrot and simmer for 5 minutes. Taste and adjust seasonings if necessary.

5. Spoon mixture into an ovenproof casserole, sprinkle top with bread crumbs and bake for about 15 minutes or until fish is cooked through and casserole is bubbly. Serve immediately.

SERVES 4

Per serving: 285 calories; 22.0 grams protein; 39.5 grams carbohydrates; 4.6 grams fat (1.7 grams fat from fish); 29 milligrams cholesterol; 160 milligrams sodium (without salting).

# CASSEROLE OF RED SNAPPER WITH SPINACH AND POTATOES

This is my rendition of a Basque favorite—minus the oodles of oil, sausages, and other enemies of the heart and arteries found in the original. A complete dinner, it needs no more accompaniment than some good, crusty bread.

2 teaspoons olive oil
1 small onion, minced
2 cloves garlic, pressed
4 ripe tomatoes, peeled and chopped
1/2 cup dry white wine
1/2 cup chopped fresh basil or parsley
1/2 cup Low Fat Chicken Stock (page 3) or canned low
  sodium broth
3 medium potatoes, peeled, quartered, and cooked
10 ounces cooked spinach, drained and chopped
  Salt and freshly ground pepper to taste
1 pound red snapper fillets
1/2 teaspoon dried thyme

1. Preheat oven to 350° F.
2. Heat oil in a medium saucepan. Add onion and garlic and cook over low heat, stirring, for 1 minute. Add tomatoes and wine, cover, and cook for 10 minutes. Stir in basil.
3. While tomato mixture simmers, heat stock in another medium saucepan. Remove from heat. Add

potatoes and spinach, and mash until thoroughly combined. Season to taste with salt and pepper.

4. Spoon half of tomato sauce mixture over the bottom of an ovenproof casserole. Top with half of potato-spinach mixture. Place red snapper on top and season with thyme. Top with remainder of tomato sauce, and finish with layer of potato-spinach combination. Cover casserole and bake for 30 minutes.

SERVES 4

Per serving: 275 calories; 29.5 grams protein; 28.5 grams carbohydrates; 4.8 grams fat (1.5 grams fat from fish); 42 milligrams cholesterol; 185 milligrams sodium (without salting).

# WHITEFISH LAYERED WITH POTATO AND SWEET PEPPERS

Surprising filling, I would follow this dish with a lovely fruit dessert, such as fresh fruit salad, fruit compote, or whole skinned pears seeped in spiced wine.

    *Vegetable oil cooking spray*
  1 *tablespoon fine bread crumbs*
1¼ *pounds whitefish fillets*
  1 *teaspoon medium-hot paprika or freshly ground*
      *pepper*
  4 *medium potatoes, halved and parboiled*
  2 *medium green bell peppers, cut into ¹/₂-inch rings*
  2 *medium tomatoes, sliced*
¹/₄ *cup low fat (1%) milk*
¹/₂ *cup light sour cream*

1. Preheat oven to 375° F.

2. Coat a casserole or ovenproof casserole or baking dish with vegetable oil cooking spray. Sprinkle with bread crumbs.

3. Season fish with paprika or ground pepper and set aside.

4. Peel cooked potatoes and cut into ¹/₂-inch slices. Arrange potatoes on bottom of prepared casserole or baking dish. Place pepper rings over potatoes, and

top with tomato slices. Arrange fish fillets over vegetables, cover, and bake for 10 minutes.

5. Combine milk and sour cream in a small bowl. Mix well and spoon over fish. Bake, uncovered, for an additional 20 minutes or until potatoes are tender and fish is cooked. Baste fish every 10 minutes with liquid from baking dish.

SERVES 4

Per serving: 340 calories; 33.0 grams protein; 27.5 grams carbohydrates; 11.0 grams fat (8.7 grams fat from fish); 90 milligrams cholesterol; 125 milligrams sodium (without salting).

# HADDOCK BAKED
# ON A BED OF VEGETABLES

Here is a savory recipe that's really low in calories to add to your repertoire of dinners-in-a-dish.

  1 lemon
  6 stalks celery, thinly sliced
  1 large onion, cut into rings
  1 large potato, peeled and cut into small cubes
  1/2 teaspoon dried oregano
  1 cup dry white wine
  1 cup Low Fat Chicken Stock (page 3) or canned low
       sodium broth
    Salt and freshly ground pepper to taste
  4 haddock fillets, about 5 ounces each
  2 teaspoons olive oil

1. Using a vegetable peeler or lemon zester, peel lemon. Cut peel into thin strips. Cut lemon in half and press out juice, discarding seeds and shell.

2. In a medium saucepan, combine lemon peel and juice with celery, onion, potato, oregano, wine, stock, and salt and pepper. Bring to a simmer, then cover and cook over low heat for about 15 minutes or until potato is almost tender.

3. Meanwhile, preheat oven to 400° F.

4. Transfer vegetables and liquid from saucepan to an ovenproof casserole or baking dish large enough to hold the fish in one layer. Place fish fillets on top

of vegetables. Drizzle oil over fish, cover with foil, and bake for about 10 minutes or until fish is cooked through and potato is tender. Uncover casserole and serve.

SERVES 4

Per serving: 235 calories; 29.0 grams protein; 21.0 grams carbohydrates; 4.0 grams fat (1.0 gram fat from fish); 82 milligrams cholesterol; 175 milligrams sodium (without salting).

# CATFISH AND
# SPAGHETTI SQUASH
# IN CREAMY TOMATO SAUCE

Don't be turned off by the amount of ingredients in this recipe—read through the steps of preparation and you'll see how easily they all come together. This will also give you some notion of how attractive this unusual dish will be and how splendid it will taste.

  *1 spaghetti squash, about 2 pounds*
  *1 cup Low Fat Chicken Stock (page 3) or canned low
      sodium broth*
  *2 teaspoons vegetable oil*
  *2 small zucchini, diced*
  *6 ounces mushrooms, wiped clean and diced*
  *1 clove garlic, pressed*
  *6 scallions, whites and tender greens, chopped*
  *2 tablespoons minced fresh basil or parsley*
  *1 teaspoon dried oregano*
  *Salt and freshly ground pepper to taste*
  *1 pound catfish fillets, cut into 1-inch pieces*
  *1/4 cup evaporated low fat milk*
  *1/2 cup canned no-salt-added tomato sauce*
  *1 tablespoon fine flour*
  *1 cup bread crumbs, made from 2 slices dried firm
      white bread*

1. Preheat oven to 350° F.

2. Slash squash in several places, place on a baking sheet, and bake for 45 minutes to 1 hour or until squash can be easily pierced with fork.

3. While squash bakes, heat stock and oil in a large skillet. When simmering, add zucchini, mushrooms, and garlic and cook over medium heat, stirring frequently, for 5 minutes. Stir in scallions, basil, oregano, salt and pepper to taste, and cook for an additional 2 minutes or until vegetables are just tender. Remove from heat.

4. When squash is cooked, remove from oven and let cool slightly. Do not turn off oven. Cut squash in half lengthwise and remove seeds. Using a fork, scrape pulp into a shallow baking pan or ovenproof casserole, smoothing top. Cover squash with catfish, then spoon zucchini-mushroom mixture and contents of skillet over fish.

5. Combine milk and tomato sauce in a small bowl and stir in flour until blended. Pour mixture into baking pan. Sprinkle top with bread crumbs and bake in hot oven for about 20 minutes or until bubbly. Serve immediately.

SERVES 4
Per serving: 300 calories; 26.5 grams protein; 27.5 grams carbohydrates; 9.5 grams fat (4.8 grams fat from fish); 66 milligrams cholesterol; 225 milligrams sodium (without salting).

# SHRIMP-STUFFED FLOUNDER

In this recipe, half the flounder fillets are spread over the bottom of a shallow casserole, then covered with a delicious shrimp- and mushroom-based filling and topped with the other half of the fillets. I often think of this as a grand baked flounder sandwich. Good with asparagus served either hot or at room temperature.

Vegetable oil cooking spray
1 tablespoon vegetable oil
4 large shallots, minced
2 stalks celery, chopped
6 medium mushrooms, wiped clean and chopped
1/4 pound shrimp, shelled, deveined, and chopped
1 tablespoon minced fresh parsley or 1/2 tablespoon dried
1/2 cup dry white wine
1 cup Low Fat Chicken Stock (page 3) or canned low sodium broth
Salt and freshly ground pepper to taste
1 tablespoon fine flour
1 pound flounder fillets
1/2 cup fine bread crumbs, made from 1 slice dried firm white bread

1. Preheat oven to 375° F. Lightly coat a shallow casserole or baking dish with cooking spray and set aside.

2. Heat oil in a large nonstick skillet. Add shallots, celery, and mushrooms. Cook over medium-low heat, stirring, for 2 minutes. Cover and simmer gently for an additional 2 minutes. Add shrimp and parsley and stir for 2 minutes. Remove skillet from heat.

3. Bring wine and stock to a simmer in a small saucepan. Season with salt and pepper, and stir in flour. Simmer gently, stirring, for about 1 minute or until mixture thickens.

4. Spread half the flounder fillets over bottom of prepared casserole or baking pan. Spoon contents from skillet over flounder, then cover with remaining fillets. Spoon contents from saucepan over all and sprinkle with bread crumbs. Cover with foil and bake for 10 minutes, then remove foil and bake an additional 5 minutes or until bubbly and cooked through.

SERVES 4

Per serving: 230 calories; 29.5 grams protein; 13.5 grams carbohydrates; 6.7 grams fat (1.4 grams fat from fish); 98 milligrams cholesterol; 215 milligrams sodium (without salting).

# THE MAIN COURSE:
# BRAISED AND LIGHTLY SAUTÉED

# SAUTÉED COD
# WITH ROASTED PEPPER SAUCE

Quickly sautéed cod is a perfect match for this stunning roasted red pepper sauce, which may serve either as a bed or topping for the fish. The sauce can be prepared in advance and refrigerated, covered, for up to 24 hours, then gently reheated just before serving.

> 1 large red bell pepper
> ½ cup Low Fat Chicken Stock (page 3) or canned low sodium broth
> Pinch cayenne pepper or to taste
> 1 tablespoon olive oil
> 4 cod fillets, each about 5 ounces
> Salt and freshly ground pepper to taste
> 1 cup shredded daikon (Asian radish) or white icicle radish

1. Roast red pepper by charring skin on all sides under broiler or over gas flame. Place blackened pepper in a paper bag. Close bag, allowing pepper to steam, and let stand until cool enough to handle. Peel off charred skin (easiest done with wet hands), then core and seed pepper. Cut into pieces and place in a food processor. Add stock and cayenne, and process until smoothly pureed. Spoon into a small bowl and set aside.

2. Heat oil in a large nonstick skillet. Add cod and

cook over medium heat for 4 to 5 minutes on each side or until fish is lightly browned and cooked through. Season to taste with salt and pepper.

3. Transfer fish to a heated serving platter or individual plates. Spoon red pepper sauce over each fillet and serve garnished with shredded radish.

SERVES 4

Per serving: 165 calories; 26.5 grams protein; 3.5 grams carbohydrates; 4.7 grams fat (1.0 gram fat from fish); 62 milligrams cholesterol; 95 milligrams sodium (without salting).

# MAKO SHARK
# WITH MUSHROOMS AND
# RADICCHIO

The headline should read "Man Bites Shark—And Begs for More." Delicious mako shark is found in the Gulf of Mexico and on both the Atlantic and Pacific coasts. It can grow up to 12 feet long and weigh as much as 200 pounds. Mako flesh is very lean and does not need a long cooking time, so keep a watchful eye when preparing the fillets to make certain they're not overdone.

*1/2 pound mushrooms, with stems, wiped clean and thickly sliced*

*1 clove garlic, minced*

*1 tablespoon white wine*

*1/2 cup Low Fat Chicken Stock (page 3) or canned low sodium broth*

*1/4 teaspoon hot paprika or to taste*

*4 mako shark fillets, about 5 ounces each*

*2 teaspoons cracked black peppercorns*

*1/2 tablespoon olive or vegetable oil*

*1 small head radicchio, separated into leaves, each leaf broken into 3 to 4 pieces*

1. Combine mushrooms, garlic, wine, 1/4 cup stock, and paprika in a medium saucepan. Cover and cook over low heat for 8 to 10 minutes or until

mushrooms are tender. Remove from heat and set aside.

2. Meanwhile, roll fish fillets in cracked pepper, using your hands to press pepper into fish.

3. Heat oil in a nonstick skillet large enough to hold fish in one layer. Add fish and brown, uncovered, on both sides. Mako is very lean; be careful not to overcook; depending on thickness of fish, 4 minutes on each side should do it. Remove fish from skillet and keep warm. Add remaining stock to skillet and bring to a simmer.

4. Arrange radicchio on a serving platter. Place fish fillets on lettuce and spoon mushrooms and contents of saucepan over fish. Top all with sauce from skillet and serve at once.

SERVES 4

Per serving: 225 calories; 31.5 grams protein; 5.5 grams carbohydrates; 8.7 grams fat (6.5 grams fat from fish); 73 milligrams cholesterol; 125 milligrams sodium (without salting).

# HONEYED SALMON SAUTÉ

The marinade lends a hot, sweet and sour quality to the salmon so that the resulting product has a lively barbecue sauciness. Good accompaniments include whipped potatoes and/or stir-fried cabbage.

  *4 teaspoons honey*
  *1 tablespoon Worcestershire sauce*
  *¼ cup Low Fat Chicken Stock (page 3) or canned low sodium broth*
  *¼ teaspoon hot pepper sauce or to taste*
  *1 pound salmon fillets*
  *1 tablespoon olive oil*

1. Combine honey, Worcestershire sauce, stock, and hot pepper sauce in a small bowl. Mix thoroughly.

2. Place salmon fillets in a shallow dish and spoon honey mixture over fish. Marinate for 20 minutes, turning fish twice. Do not refrigerate.

3. Heat oil in a large nonstick skillet. Add fish and sauté over high heat for 3 to 5 minutes on each side, depending on thickness of fish. Transfer fish to a heated platter or dinner plates and serve.

Per serving: 215 calories; 23.0 grams protein; 6.5 grams carbohydrates; 10.8 grams fat (7.2 grams fat from fish); 62 milligrams cholesterol; 100 milligrams sodium (without salting).

# FILLET OF FLUKE
# WITH LIME AND CUMIN

This recipe calls for fluke fillets quickly braised in a stock seasoned with garlic, hot pepper flakes, cumin, coriander, turmeric, soy sauce, and lime juice. Redolent of flavorings and aromas, try it with any simply steamed vegetable.

Vegetable oil cooking spray
$1/3$ cup Fish Stock (page 5) or canned low sodium broth
$1^1/4$ pounds fluke fillets
1 clove garlic, pressed
$1/4$ teaspoon hot red pepper flakes
1 teaspoon ground cumin or to taste
$1/2$ teaspoon coriander seeds
$1/2$ teaspoon ground turmeric
2 teaspoons low sodium soy sauce
Juice of 2 limes
1 lime, thinly sliced

1. Coat a large skillet with vegetable oil cooking spray. Add stock and heat. Place fish in skillet, baste with stock, cover, and cook for 4 minutes. Carefully transfer fish to a platter and keep warm.

2. Add all remaining ingredients, except lime juice and slices, to skillet and cook over medium-high heat, stirring, for 1 minute.

3. Return fish to skillet and add lime juice. Baste fish with warm sauce and simmer until cooked

through. Transfer fish to a serving dish, spoon sauce over all, garnish with lime slices and serve.

SERVES 4

Per serving: 205 calories; 27.5 grams protein; 2.5 grams carbohydrates; 9.4 grams fat (8.4 grams fat from fish); 85 milligrams cholesterol; 190 milligrams sodium (without salting).

# SWORDFISH KANSAS CITY STYLE

This sauce, made with cider vinegar, ketchup, Worcestershire, and hot pepper sauce is reminiscent of the kind served in K.C. over barbecued meat. It has only a fraction of the fat but boasts enough bravado to stand up to "meaty" swordfish steaks.

Red and white cabbage slaw, boiled new potatoes, or corn-on-the-cob would be perfect on the side.

 4 teaspoons vegetable or peanut oil
 2 tablespoons cider vinegar
 1/4 cup low sodium ketchup
 2 teaspoons Worcestershire sauce
 1/2 teaspoon hot pepper sauce or to taste
 1 pound swordfish steaks

1. Combine 2 teaspoons oil, vinegar, ketchup, Worcestershire sauce, and hot pepper sauce in a small saucepan. Bring to a simmer, stirring, and remove from heat and set aside.

2. Heat remaining 2 teaspoons oil in a large nonstick skillet. Place fish steaks in skillet and sauté over medium-high heat for 3 to 4 minutes on each side, or until fish is cooked through.

3. Carefully transfer swordfish to a large, shallow pan. Pour reserved sauce over fish and allow to mar-

inate for 30 minutes. Serve swordfish with its marinade at room temperature.

SERVES 4
Per serving: 200 calories; 23.0 grams protein; 5.0 grams carbohydrates; 9.5 grams fat (4.6 grams fat from fish); 45 milligrams cholesterol; 145 milligrams sodium (without salting).

# BROOK TROUT WITH APPLE-HORSERADISH SAUCE

The mild, sweet flesh of trout makes them a favorite on the grill or skillet, and their moderate to high fat content makes them desirable to those of us interested in the remarkable benefits attributed to Omega-3.

This simple recipe brings out the best in the trout, but my apple-yogurt-horseradish troika elevates this dish to the sublime.

1 Granny Smith or other tart apple, peeled, cored, and grated
4 tablespoons nonfat plain yogurt
4 tablespoons prepared horseradish, liquid pressed out
4 whole brook trout, about 8 ounces each, cleaned and trimmed to taste
1/4 cup flour
Salt and freshly ground pepper to taste
1 tablespoon vegetable or olive oil

1. Combine apple, yogurt, and horseradish in a small bowl. Mix until thoroughly blended and refrigerate for about 1 hour.

2. Dredge trout in flour combined with salt and pepper to taste. Shake off excess flour.

3. Heat oil in a nonstick skillet large enough to hold all the trout in one layer. Add trout to skillet and cook over medium-high heat for 5 minutes on

one side. Turn and cook on other side for about 6 minutes or until trout is cooked through and lightly browned.

4. Transfer trout to individual plates and serve hot with chilled apple-horseradish sauce on the side.

SERVES 4
Per serving: 255 calories; 25.0 grams protein; 12.0 grams carbohydrates; 11.4 grams fat (7.5 grams fat from fish); 67 milligrams cholesterol; 210 milligrams sodium (without salting).

# GROUPER BRAISED IN
# CHAMPAGNE
# WITH FRESH GRAPES

The French call dishes garnished with grapes *Véronique*. And my growing list of favorite dishes *Véronique* is headed by the low fat recipe I've devised for the sweet-flavored grouper. Here, the fish is filmed with flour, quickly browned, then braised in a gentle bath of stock and champagne. I prefer a combination of green and red seedless grapes for this preparation because it adds a more interesting color contrast, but either will work alone.

   1 pound grouper fillets
   3 tablespoons all-purpose flour
      Salt and freshly ground pepper to taste
   1 tablespoon olive oil
   6 scallions, white part only, minced
   1/2 cup Low Fat Chicken Stock (page 3) or low sodium broth
   3/4 cup champagne or dry white wine
   1 1/2 cups green or red (or combination) seedless grapes, cut in half

1. Dredge fish in flour combined with salt and pepper. Shake off excess and set aside.
2. Heat oil in a large nonstick skillet. Add scallions and cook over low heat, stirring, for 1 minute. Raise

heat to medium high. Add fish and cook for 3 minutes. Turn fish to other side.

3. Add stock and $1/2$ cup of the champagne to fish in skillet and bring to a boil. Reduce heat to low and simmer, spooning liquid from skillet over fish frequently, for 5 minutes or until fish is cooked through. Carefully transfer fish to a heated serving platter.

4. Add remaining champagne and the grapes to skillet and bring to a boil. Stir over medium-high heat for about 3 minutes or until grapes are very hot and sauce is bubbly. Spoon sauce and grapes over fish and serve.

SERVES 4

Per serving: 190 calories; 23.0 grams protein; 12.5 grams carbohydrates; 5.0 grams fat (1.2 grams fat from fish); 42 milligrams cholesterol; 75 milligrams sodium (without salting).

# BRAISED YELLOWTAIL WITH APPLES AND SESAME SEEDS

This recipe is quick and easy, practically oil-free, and works with most delicately flavored fillets. Simple yet luscious, serve and wait for the compliments.

*1 medium golden delicious apple, unpeeled, cored, and cut into 8 wedges*
*1 cup apple juice*
*2 teaspoons fresh lemon juice*
*Olive oil cooking spray*
*2 large shallots, thinly sliced*
*1 stalk celery, thinly sliced*
*1¼ pounds yellowtail fillets (or tuna steaks)*
*Salt and freshly ground pepper to taste*
*1½ tablespoons toasted sesame seeds*

1. Combine apple with ½ cup apple juice and lemon juice in a small saucepan. Cover and cook over low heat until apples are barely tender. Remove from heat and set aside.

2. Coat a large nonstick skillet with cooking spray. Add shallots and celery and cook, stirring, for 2 minutes.

3. Place fish in skillet. Add remaining ½ cup apple juice and cover. Cook for about 5 minutes or until

fish is cooked through. Transfer fish to a serving platter and keep warm.

4. Pour skillet contents into saucepan containing apple wedges. Heat and pour over fish. Sprinkle with sesame seeds and serve.

SERVES 4

Per serving: 290 calories; 34.0 grams protein; 15.5 grams carbohydrates; 10.2 grams fat (7.5 grams fat from fish); 54 milligrams cholesterol; 70 milligrams sodium (without salting).

# BAY SCALLOPS
# IN SPICED MUSTARD SAUCE

This recipe for bay scallops is another example of taste without guilt. An even-handed coating of coriander, paprika, turmeric, and cumin gives the scallops a certain zest. They are then lightly sautéed with scallions and bathed in a reduced sauce of stock, wine, and mustard to create a gentle explosion calculated to excite the taste buds.

Noodles would be perfect alongside this dish.

$1^1/_2$ teaspoons ground coriander
1 teaspoon mild or hot paprika
1 teaspoon ground turmeric
$^1/_2$ teaspoon ground cumin
   Salt and freshly ground pepper to taste
1 pound bay scallops (or sea scallops quartered),
   rinsed and patted dry
1 tablespoon peanut or vegetable oil
1 large clove garlic, minced
6 scallions, white and tender greens, chopped
$^1/_2$ cup Low Fat Chicken Stock (page 3) or canned low
   sodium broth
$^1/_4$ cup dry white wine
1 tablespoon Dijon mustard or to taste

1. In a mixing bowl, combine spices and seasonings and stir well. Add scallops and toss to coat with spices. Let stand for 10 minutes.

2. Heat oil in a large nonstick skillet. Add garlic and scallions and stir over high heat for 2 minutes. Reduce heat to medium.

3. Add scallops to skillet and cook, stirring frequently, for 2 minutes. Using a slotted spoon, remove scallops from skillet and set aside.

4. Add stock, wine, and mustard to scallions in skillet and stir to blend. Bring to a boil, then reduce heat to medium and simmer for 2 minutes or until liquid is reduced by a third.

5. Return scallops to skillet and cook, gently stirring to coat them with the sauce, for 2 to 3 minutes or until cooked through. Serve hot.

SERVES 4

Per serving: 150 calories; 20.0 grams protein; 5.5 grams carbohydrates; 5.0 grams fat (.9 gram fat from fish); 38 milligrams cholesterol; 315 milligrams sodium (without salting).

# SEA SCALLOPS
# WITH WILD MUSHROOMS

So outrageously good is this dish, you may have a tough time parting with any. But the praise you're sure to receive is well worth your generosity. Use the wild mushroom mix of your choice, but please do not use the white button (cultivated) mushrooms for this recipe; it will definitely not taste the same.

Asparagus makes a worthy accompaniment, as would a salad of arugula, watercress, or dandelion greens.

*1/2 pound fresh wild mushrooms (oyster, chanterelle,*
*morels, portobello, etc., or any combination),*
*wiped clean, trimmed, and sliced*
*1 1/2 cups Low Fat Chicken Stock (page 3) or canned low*
*sodium broth*
*1 pound sea scallops*
*1 tablespoon olive oil*
*Salt and freshly ground pepper to taste*
*2 tablespoons chopped fresh chives*

1. Combine mushrooms and stock in a medium saucepan. Cook over medium heat until mushrooms are tender and liquid has been reduced by half.

2. Wash scallops, cut in half horizontally, and pat dry.

3. Heat olive oil in a large nonstick skillet. Add

scallops and cook over medium-high heat, tossing to brown them slightly on both sides. Do not overcook. Scallops should be done in 2 to 3 minutes. Using a slotted spoon, transfer scallops to a heated serving platter and keep warm.

4. Add mushrooms and sauce to skillet, season to taste with salt and pepper and heat to a simmer.

5. Spoon mushrooms and sauce from skillet onto scallops, sprinkle top with chives, and serve.

SERVES 4

Per serving: 155 calories; 20.5 grams protein; 6.5 grams carbohydrates; 5.0 grams fat (.9 gram fat from fish); 39 milligrams cholesterol; 210 milligrams sodium (without salting).

# BUTTERFLY SHRIMP
# SAUTÉED WITH JALAPEÑOS

Bring a bit of the Southwest to your dining table with this flavorful creation. But, remember: jalapeños can be very hot! If you can't stand too much heat, use just one jalapeño pepper.

Chill out with any plain rice, potato, or pasta preparation.

1 pound large shrimp, rinsed, shelled, and deveined
2 tablespoons flour
Olive oil cooking spray
4 cloves garlic, pressed
2 small jalapeño peppers, cored, seeded, and minced
(wear gloves)
$\frac{1}{2}$ cup Low Fat Chicken Stock (page 3) or canned low
sodium broth
Salt to taste
$\frac{1}{4}$ head chicory lettuce, separated into leaves

1. To butterfly shrimp, cut them lengthwise in half, being very careful not to cut through to other side. Gently spread shrimp halves to form butterfly shape. Dust lightly with flour and set aside.

2. Coat a large nonstick skillet with cooking spray. Add garlic and stir over medium heat for 1 minute. Add jalapeños, stock, and salt and continue cooking, stirring, for 2 minutes.

3. Turn heat to high and add shrimp. Cook, turn-

ing shrimp from side to side for 4 to 5 minutes or until shrimp are pink and cooked through.

4. Place chicory on a platter, top with shrimp and contents of skillet, and serve.

SERVES 4

Per serving: 150 calories; 24.0 grams protein; 7.0 grams carbohydrates; 2.9 grams fat (2.0 grams fat from fish); 173 milligrams cholesterol; 195 milligrams sodium (without salting).

# SAUTÉED SOFT-SHELL CRABS

Soft-shell crab is a blue crab just after molting, when it has emerged from its hard back and has only a soft shell. It is completely edible, save its face and gills, and ranges from about 3 to 6 inches. In my opinion, the smaller the better.

I love to make a lunch of this tarragon-scented dish, with just a simple salad of field greens or, for heartier appetites, fresh corn.

*8 soft-shell crabs, about 3 ounces each, cleaned*
*1 cup low fat (2%) milk*
*4 tablespoons all-purpose flour*
*¾ teaspoon dried tarragon*
  *Salt and freshly ground pepper to taste*
*1 tablespoon peanut or vegetable oil*
*2 lemons, each cut into 4 wedges*

1. Place crabs in a large shallow pan. Pour milk over crabs and allow to marinate in milk for 20 minutes, turning crabs twice.

2. Combine flour with tarragon and salt and pepper to taste and spread on a large, flat plate. Remove crabs from milk. Dredge crabs in flour mixture and shake off excess flour.

3. Heat oil in a large nonstick skillet. Add crabs and sauté for 3 to 4 minutes on each side or until cooked through. Remove crabs as they cook to a

serving platter and keep warm. Garnish with lemon wedges.

SERVES 4

Per serving: 225 calories; 28.0 grams protein; 14.0 grams carbohydrates; 6.4 grams fat (1.5 grams fat from fish); 115 milligrams cholesterol; 450 milligrams sodium (without salting).

# LEMON-BRAISED SEA BASS WITH FENNEL

This fennel mixture seems to have a natural affinity to sea bass—bringing out, rather than muzzling, its inherent flavor. The fennel is sweeter and more delicate than in its raw state, the flavor becoming even lighter and more elusive.

> 1 cup Low Fat Chicken Stock (page 3) or canned low sodium broth
> 1 fennel bulb, trimmed, rinsed, and cut vertically into thin slices
> 1/2 teaspoon dried thyme
> 1/4 teaspoon hot red pepper flakes or to taste
> 1 tablespoon margarine
> 1/3 cup dry white wine
> 2 lemons, thinly sliced
> 1 pound sea bass fillets
> Salt and freshly ground pepper to taste
> 2 teaspoons fine flour

1. Heat 1/3 cup of stock in a small saucepan. Add fennel, thyme, and hot pepper flakes. Cover and cook over low heat for about 20 minutes or until fennel is tender. Remove from heat and set aside.

2. While fennel cooks, heat margarine with remaining stock and wine in a nonstick skillet large enough to hold all the fish fillets in one layer. Add

half the lemon slices and simmer, uncovered, over medium heat for 2 minutes.

3. Place fish in skillet and season to taste with salt and pepper. Continue to simmer, frequently spooning skillet liquid over fish, for about 8 minutes or until fish is cooked through.

4. Using a slotted spatula, transfer fish to a serving platter and keep warm.

5. Remove lemon slices from skillet and discard. Add fennel with contents from saucepan to skillet and bring to a boil. Sprinkle flour into skillet and stir over medium heat until thoroughly blended and sauce is slightly thickened. Spoon fennel and sauce over fish and serve on a large platter garnished with remaining lemon slices.

SERVES 4
Per serving: 170 calories; 22.0 grams protein; 9.0 grams carbohydrates; 5.4 grams fat (2.3 grams fat from fish); 47 milligrams cholesterol; 150 milligrams sodium (without salting).

# FISH KOFTA BOMBAY

This Middle Eastern/Indian favorite is traditionally made with ground fatty lamb, onions, garlic, and other seasonings, and fried in a half cup or more of fat. It's then usually doused in either a rich, creamy sauce or an unctuous and rather fiery chili sauce—or both.

My version of this highly flavored dish combines fish, vegetables, and tasty Indian seasonings to produce a wonderfully exotic compound. The peas and currants that dapple the intriguing sauce add interesting texture and color contrast to this lowered fat and lowered calorie dish.

Fish Kofta

1½ pounds fish fillets (haddock, flounder, pollack, etc.), skinned and cut into pieces
1 large onion, coarsely chopped
1 large carrot, cut into pieces
2 tablespoons chopped fresh cilantro
1 teaspoon ground ginger
1 teaspoon ground turmeric
2 teaspoons cornstarch

Sauce

1 tablespoon peanut or vegetable oil
1 medium onion, chopped
2 stalks celery, cut in half lengthwise and sliced

2 cloves garlic, minced
1 large can (28 ounces) no-salt-added crushed
     tomatoes
1/2 teaspoon hot chili paste or pepper sauce or to taste
2 tablespoons finely chopped fresh cilantro
1 teaspoon each: dried turmeric, cumin, and
     cardamom
1 bay leaf
1/2 cup dried currants
1 1/2 cups fresh or frozen and thawed green peas

1. Combine all kofta ingredients in a food processor and process until coarsely pureed. Transfer to a mixing bowl. With wet hands, form mixture into small balls, about 1 1/2-inch diameter (there should be about 20 balls). Set aside.

2. To prepare sauce, heat oil in a large, deep nonstick skillet or saucepan. Add onion, celery, and garlic and cook over medium heat, stirring frequently, for 3 minutes or until softened. Add remaining sauce ingredients and bring to a simmer. Reduce heat to low and simmer gently, stirring occasionally, for 10 minutes.

3. Add fish balls to skillet, along with currants. Stir to blend, cover and simmer over low heat for 5 minutes. Add peas and simmer an additional 3 to 5 minutes or until fish is cooked through. Taste and adjust seasonings, if needed. Remove bay leaf, transfer to a heated platter or bowl, and serve.

Per serving: 255 calories; 25.5 grams protein; 29.5 grams carbohydrates; 4.0 grams fat (.8 gram fat from fish); 65 milligrams cholesterol; 135 milligrams sodium (without salting).

# WEAKFISH IN WHITE WINE WITH TOASTED ALMONDS

Also known as sea trout and gray trout, the weakfish's name comes from its weak mouth, which rips easily when released from a fishing hook. It has a fine, delicate flavor similar to brook trout and stands up well to spicy sauces. Snapper, salmon, and trout make fine substitutes.

In this recipe, weakfish is joined by a strong cast of supporting players, including the highly nutritious almond. Almonds, I am pleased to report, contain more calcium than any other nut. They also boast a very high dietary fiber content, supplying 3 grams per ounce!

  $^1/_4$ cup slivered almonds
  1 pound weakfish fillets
  1 cup dry white wine
  1 cup Fish Stock (page 5)
  1 bay leaf
  $^1/_8$ teaspoon dried marjoram
  1 clove garlic
    Pinch of crushed saffron or to taste
    Salt and freshly ground pepper to taste
  1 tablespoon chopped fresh parsley

1. Preheat oven to 300° F.
2. Place almonds on a nonstick baking sheet and

bake until nuts are a pale gold. Be careful not to burn the almonds.

3. While almonds bake, place fish in a skillet large enough to hold fish in one layer. Add wine, stock, bay leaf, marjoram, garlic, saffron, and salt and pepper. Cover and bring to a simmer. Cook about 8 minutes or until fish is cooked through.

4. Using a slotted spatula carefully transfer fish to a heated serving platter. Strain liquid from skillet and spoon over fish. Top with almonds, sprinkle with parsley, and serve.

SERVES 4
Per serving: 185 calories; 21.0 grams protein; 6.0 grams carbohydrates; 8.6 grams fat (4.1 grams fat from fish); 94 milligrams cholesterol; 90 milligrams sodium (without salting).

# THE MAIN COURSE:
# BROILED
# AND GRILLED

# SWORDFISH
# AND BABY EGGPLANT
# GRILLED EN BROCHETTE

This recipe uses baby eggplant, which has very few seeds. Depending upon your market, you may find pale lavender Chinese or Japanese eggplant, or deeply purple Italian eggplant. Whichever variety, the eggplant must be small—four will equal about one pound. You may wish to augment or substitute the eggplant with cherry tomatoes, small white boiling onions, and sweet red or green peppers. But whatever the ingredients, the technique for cooking skewered food is simple. In preparing this dish, mixing the tasty marinade and threading the skewers will be the most energetic operations you'll face.

Swordfish is lean and cooks quickly. Start with a hot grill, or if it's the wrong time of the year for outdoor cooking, prepare this dish in a preheated broiler.

*1¼ pounds swordfish steak, cut into 3-inch cubes*
*1 tablespoon balsamic vinegar*
*1 tablespoon fresh lemon juice*
*1 tablespoon dry sherry (not cooking wine)*
*1 teaspoon ground ginger*
*1 teaspoon olive oil*
*4 baby eggplant, about 1 pound total, stems removed
    and cut into large chunks*
*Mild or sweet paprika*

1. Prepare grill or preheat broiler.

2. Place fish cubes in a shallow pan. Combine vinegar, lemon juice, wine, ginger, and olive oil in a small bowl. Mix thoroughly and pour over fish. Let fish marinate for 20 minutes at room temperature, turning once or twice in marinade.

3. Thread swordfish and eggplant on four metal skewers. Brush with marinade and sprinkle with paprika. Place skewers on grill or broiler pan. Cook for 3 to 4 minutes. Turn and cook an additional 3 to 4 minutes or until fish is browned and cooked through.

SERVES 4

Per serving: 210 calories; 29.5 grams protein; 6.5 grams carbohydrates; 7.1 grams fat (5.8 grams fat from fish); 56 milligrams cholesterol; 135 milligrams sodium (without salting).

# BROILED SWORDFISH WITH HERBED ANCHOVY SAUCE

This sauce is fabulous over swordfish, but don't stop there. It complements any full-bodied fish, such as tuna. And if there is any leftover sauce, which is doubtful, it makes a scrumptious dip for fresh-toasted bread or crudités. Serve with steamed carrots and a salad of escarole.

1 swordfish steak, about 1 1/4 pounds
2 teaspoons olive oil
2 tablespoons fresh lemon juice
1/2 cup packed fresh basil leaves
1/2 cup packed fresh dill weed
2 cloves garlic
4 rolled fillet of anchovy with capers, rinsed and patted dry
2 tablespoons dry white wine

1. Preheat broiler to high.
2. Place tuna steak on a broiler pan or tray and brush with oil. Sprinkle lemon juice over fish and broil about 5 inches from heat for 5 minutes, or until brown. Turn fish carefully, and broil on second side for additional 5 minutes or until fish is done.
3. Combine all remaining ingredients in a food processor and puree.
4. Remove fish from broiler and place on a serving platter. Spread sauce over fish and serve.

Per serving: 210 calories; 30.0 grams protein; 2.5 grams carbohydrates; 8.7 grams fat (5.8 grams fat from fish); 56 milligrams cholesterol; 300 milligrams sodium (without salting).

# BROILED SHRIMP
# IN CURRY SAUCE

I serve this dish frequently using shrimp or scallops. The curry is so subtle and aromatic it gently
infuses the shrimp without overpowering its flavor. The apples add a wonderful texture and tart-
ness. Serve with rice and Cucumber Sauce (page 9)
on the side.

 3 teaspoons olive oil
 1 small onion, minced
 2 small tart apples, peeled, cored, and finely chopped
 1 clove garlic, pressed
1½ tablespoons curry powder or to taste
 1 cup Low Fat Chicken Stock (page 3) or canned low
     sodium broth
 ½ cup nonfat plain yogurt
 ¾ pound medium shrimp, shelled and deveined
     Salt and freshly ground pepper to taste
     Paprika to taste

1. Heat 1 teaspoon of the oil in a nonstick saucepan. Add onion, apples, and garlic and cook, stirring,
for 2 minutes. Add curry powder and chicken stock.
Bring to a slow simmer and cook for 5 minutes. Stir
in yogurt and simmer for an additional 2 minutes.
Dish may be prepared in advance up to this point.
Sauce may be kept warm or reheated when shrimp
are cooked.

2. Preheat broiler to high.

3. Place shrimp on a broiler pan or tray and brush with remaining oil. Season with salt, pepper, and paprika. Place shrimp about 5 inches from heat and broil about 3 minutes. Turn and broil an additional 2 minutes or until shrimp is cooked through.

4. Place shrimp on a serving platter. Heat sauce and spoon over shrimp.

SERVES 4

Per serving: 200 calories; 19.5 grams protein; 16.5 grams carbohydrates; 6.3 grams fat (1.5 grams fat from fish); 132 milligrams cholesterol; 165 milligrams sodium (without salting).

# GRILLED HALIBUT
# WITH A WALNUT COATING

Here, the cayenne pepper-laced walnut crust lends a crunchy texture to halibut and makes an excellent summer dish when the gang is coming over for a barbecue (the recipe is easily adapted for a larger group). Don't ignore this dish during the winter months, because the fish can also be wrapped in foil and baked in the oven.

   2 halibut steaks, each about 8 ounces
   3 tablespoons fresh lemon juice
     Salt to taste
  1/3 cup finely ground walnuts
   2 teaspoons peanut or vegetable oil
  1/4 teaspoon cayenne pepper or to taste


   1. Prepare grill or preheat oven to 425° F.
   2. Cut each halibut steak in half, and place each half on a sheet of heavy-duty aluminum foil. Sprinkle fish with lemon juice and salt, if desired.
   3. Combine walnuts, oil, and cayenne in a small bowl to make a paste. Spread paste over fish.
   4. Wrap foil around fish and place on barbecue grill about 3 inches from heat (or bake in oven). Grill or bake for 10 minutes. Slit top of foil to allow steam to escape, and continue cooking until fish flakes easily.

Per serving: 190 calories; 25.5 grams protein; 2.0 grams carbohydrates; 8.9 grams fat (2.6 grams fat from fish); 37 milligrams cholesterol; 60 milligrams sodium (without salting).

# MARINATED MONKFISH KEBABS

One of the best and most easily made dishes I know is this preparation of monkfish marinated and basted in an exquisite brew of stock, wine, lemon juice, fennel seeds, and cilantro. Mushrooms, pepper, and tomato are threaded alternately with the cubes of fish to round out the presentation.

Nifty with a freshly made four- or five-bean salad or uncomplicated dish of rice.

*¼ Low Fat Chicken Stock (page 3) or canned low
     sodium broth*
*¼ cup dry white wine*
*¼ cup fresh lemon juice*
*1 clove garlic, crushed*
*1 teaspoon fennel seeds*
*1 teaspoon chopped fresh cilantro*
*1¼ pounds monkfish fillet, cut into 2-inch cubes*
*8 medium mushroom caps, wiped clean*
*1 red bell pepper, cut into 8 pieces*
*8 cherry tomatoes*

1. Combine stock, wine, lemon juice, garlic, fennel seeds, and cilantro in a shallow bowl and mix well. Add fish and toss. Marinate for 1 hour, unrefrigerated, turning fish cubes in marinade every 15 minutes.

2. Prepare grill or preheat broiler.

---

3. Remove fish from marinade and reserve marinade. Thread fish cubes, alternately with mushrooms, pepper, and tomatoes on four metal skewers.

4. Place kebabs on grill or a broiler pan or tray. Grill or broil kebabs for about 15 minutes, turning and basting with marinade, until done. Serve hot.

SERVES 4

Per serving: 140 calories; 22.0 grams protein; 7.5 grams carbohydrates; 2.5 grams fat (2.1 grams fat from fish); 36 milligrams cholesterol; 40 milligrams sodium (without salting).

# FISH STEAKS
# WITH HONEY-MUSTARD GLAZE

The honey-mustard glaze adds just the right zing to this dish that works well either broiled or grilled—with tuna, salmon, or swordfish steaks.

*¼ cup dry mustard*
*2 tablespoons honey*
*2 teaspoons low sodium soy sauce*
*4 teaspoons water, approximate*
*1 pound fish steaks (tuna, swordfish, salmon)*

1. In a small bowl, combine mustard, honey, and soy sauce. Add water by the teaspoonful, stirring constantly, until mixture is smooth and thick enough to coat a spoon.

2. Brush mustard mixture on fish, coating both sides. Let marinate, unrefrigerated, for 15 minutes.

3. Prepare grill or preheat broiler.

4. Grill or broil fish about 4 inches from heat for 4 to 5 minutes on each side, depending on thickness, or until fish is just cooked through. Serve hot.

SERVES 4
Per serving: 220 calories; 28.0 grams protein; 9.5 grams carbohydrates; 7.5 grams fat (5.6 grams fat from fish); 43 milligrams cholesterol; 150 milligrams sodium (without salting).

# TUNA TERIYAKI

After marinating the sturdy fish in a mixture of dry sherry, soy sauce, a touch of sugar, and minced ginger, the fish is quickly broiled. I have eliminated the oil and opted for low sodium soy sauce, but otherwise the intense flavor—and I hope spirit—of teriyaki remains intact.

The ideal accompaniment for tuna teriyaki is steamed rice and perhaps a salad of crisp fresh bean sprouts drizzled with rice vinegar.

*½ cup dry sherry (not cooking wine)*
*¼ cup low sodium soy sauce*
*1 tablespoon sugar*
*1 large clove garlic, pressed*
*1 tablespoon finely minced peeled ginger root*
*4 tuna steaks, about 5 ounces each*

1. In a small saucepan combine sherry, soy sauce, and sugar and bring to a brisk simmer. Add garlic and ginger and stir over high heat for 1 minute. Remove from heat and let sauce cool to room temperature.

2. Place tuna steaks in a shallow glass bowl or platter. Pour cooled sauce over tuna. Cover and refrigerate for 30 minutes, turning tuna after 15 minutes. Remove from refrigerator and let stand at room temperature for an additional 30 minutes, turning once.

3. Prepare grill or preheat broiler.

4. Grill or broil tuna 4 to 5 inches from heat for about 4 minutes. Turn fish, brush with marinade and cook an additional 4 to 5 minutes or until tuna is cooked through. Transfer to a heated platter and serve.

SERVES 4

Per serving: 230 calories; 34.0 grams protein; 6.5 grams carbohydrates; 7.0 grams fat (7.0 grams fat from fish); 54 milligrams cholesterol; 540 milligrams sodium (without salting).

# BROILED SHAD WITH GRATIN OF FENNEL, ZUCCHINI, AND TOMATOES

Shad is a richly flavored fish that contains many tiny bones. The only way to purchase shad is deboned. When cooking do not attempt to turn the shad over; it's constructed with flaps of fish meat and to try to turn it is to be left with a real mess.

>     Vegetable oil cooking spray
>   1 medium fennel bulb, trimmed and chopped
>   2 medium zucchini, thinly sliced
>   4 plum tomatoes, diced
>   1 tablespoon olive oil
>   1 teaspoon balsamic vinegar
>     Salt and freshly ground pepper to taste
> 1 or 2 shad fillets, deboned, about 1¼ pounds

1. Preheat broiler. Coat a shallow, nonstick baking pan with cooking spray and set aside.

2. Combine fennel, zucchini, tomatoes, oil, and vinegar in a heavy saucepan. Season to taste with salt and pepper and cook, stirring occasionally, for 5 to 8 minutes or until vegetables are just cooked through. Remove from heat and set aside. Gratin may be made the day before, refrigerated, then served at room temperature.

3. Place shad fillets, skin-side down, in prepared

baking pan and broil for about 15 minutes or until fish flakes easily when tested at the thickest part.

4. Divide fish into 4 portions and place on heated plates. Spoon vegetable gratin beside fish and serve.

SERVES 4
Per serving: 350 calories; 26.0 grams protein; 7.5 grams carbohydrates; 24.2 grams fat (19.5 grams fat from fish); cholesterol data unavailable; 110 milligrams sodium (without salting).

# SALMON STEAKS IN SWEET GRAPEFRUIT AND WINE SAUCE

The sauce, with its sweet and tart elements, accents rather than stifles the full, rich essence of broiled salmon. This dish is given added panache by presenting the beautiful pink grapefruit segments and the sauce around the fish.

Brown rice studded with tiny peas would make a lovely accompaniment.

    2 pink grapefruits
    1/4 cup Burgundy or other fruity red wine
    1 1/2 tablespoons sugar
        Salt and freshly ground pepper to taste
    4 salmon steaks, about 5 ounces each

1. Peel and separate one of the grapefruits into segments, reserving excess juice (if any), and set aside.

2. Squeeze juice from second grapefruit and pour into a small saucepan with excess juice from first grapefruit. Add wine, sugar, and salt and pepper to grapefruit juice and bring to a boil. Reduce heat and let simmer gently, stirring occasionally, for 2 minutes. Remove from heat and let cool slightly.

3. Place salmon steaks in a shallow nonstick baking pan and spoon on half of the grapefruit sauce.

Let fish stand, unrefrigerated, for 10 minutes, turning fish once.

4. Preheat broiler.

5. Broil fish about 4 inches from heat for 4 minutes. Turn, spoon sauce from baking pan over fish and broil an additional 4 to 5 minutes or until fish is cooked through.

6. While fish broils, place reserved grapefruit segments in remaining grapefruit sauce in saucepan and simmer over very low heat for 2 minutes.

7. Transfer fish to a heated platter, spoon grapefruit sections and sauce around fish, and serve.

SERVES 4

Per serving: 255 calories; 29.0 grams protein; 14.5 grams carbohydrates; 9.1 grams fat (9.0 grams fat from fish); 78 milligrams cholesterol; 65 milligrams sodium (without salting).

# BROILED CATFISH
# IN MINTED MARINADE

This fish gets its name from the long whiskerlike feelers that hang down from around its mouth. Most catfish are freshwater fish, and the majority in today's market are farmed. The flesh is firm, mild-flavored, and takes well to the broiler.

   Juice from 1 large lemon
   1 tablespoon minced fresh mint or 1¹/₂ teaspoon dried
   ¹/₂ tablespoon minced fresh parsley or 1 teaspoon dried
   2 teaspoons olive or vegetable oil
   Olive oil cooking spray
   1 pound catfish fillets
   Salt and freshly ground pepper to taste
   Lemon slices and sprigs of fresh mint or parsley for
      garnish

1. Combine lemon juice, mint, parsley, and oil in a shallow dish and stir well. Add fish, turning to coat on all sides. Marinate at room temperature for 10 minutes.

2. While fish marinates, preheat broiler.

3. Place catfish in one layer on a broiler pan coated with cooking spray. Spoon on any excess marinade and salt and pepper. Broil fish about 5 inches from heat for about 5 minutes or until cooked through. Do not turn.

4. Transfer fish to a heated platter and serve garnished with lemon slices and mint or parsley sprigs.

SERVES 4

Per serving: 155 calories; 20.5 grams protein; .5 grams carbohydrates; 7.9 grams fat (4.8 grams fat from fish); 66 milligrams cholesterol; 75 milligrams sodium (without salting).

# THE MAIN COURSE:
# STEAMED AND POACHED

# LEMON SOLE ROLLS
# WITH DILLED YOGURT SAUCE

To make sure the rolled fillets cook evenly and will fit in the steamer basket, choose thin fillets of sole. If the fillets are thick through the center bone line, make a slit down the line with a sharp knife, being careful not to cut through the fish. If lemon sole is unavailable, substitute grey sole, flounder, farm-raised catfish, or other small thin fillets of fish. Here, the fillets are rolled around fresh minced dill weed, which is, to my mind, the herb most complementary to the delicate nature of sole. The simple vinegar-splashed, dilled yogurt sauce carries through the flavor idea and makes a lovely topping.

Accompany with just about any colorful rice or potato preparation, such as confetti rice or boiled potatoes sprinkled with paprika.

8 thin lemon sole fillets, about 1¼ pounds total
   Juice of 1 lemon
3 tablespoons minced fresh dill weed
   Salt and freshly ground pepper to taste
½ cup low fat plain yogurt
2 teaspoons white wine vinegar
   Lemon slices and dill sprigs for garnish

1. Put water to boil in a steamer with a rack.
2. While waiting for water to boil, spread fish fil-

lets side by side. Sprinkle surface with lemon juice, 1 tablespoon of the minced dill, and salt and pepper to taste. Roll up each fillet, jelly-roll fashion, and secure with a toothpick.

3. Place fish rolls on steamer rack and place in steamer. Cover as tightly as possible and steam fish for about 8 minutes or until cooked through.

4. While fish steams, combine yogurt with remaining 2 tablespoons dill and vinegar in a small saucepan and stir over very low heat for 2 minutes or until thoroughly hot and at a bare simmer.

5. Remove fish from steamer, place on a heated serving dish and remove toothpicks. Serve garnished with lemon wedges and dill sprigs and with the dilled-yogurt sauce on the side.

SERVES 4

Per serving: 150 calories; 28.5 grams protein; 3.0 grams carbohydrates; 2.2 grams fat (1.7 grams fat from fish); 70 milligrams cholesterol; 140 milligrams sodium (without salting).

# MUSSELS IN WHITE WINE
# WITH SWISS CHARD

Mussels in white wine *(moules marinière)* is a traditional and popular dish served throughout France. This version adds Swiss chard (use spinach if chard is unavailable) and diced tomatoes for a more robust sauce.

- *1 tablespoon olive oil*
- *6 shallots, minced*
- *2 cloves garlic, minced*
- *3 cups dry white wine, such as Muscadet*
- *1 bay leaf*
- *1 tablespoon chopped fresh thyme or 1 teaspoon dried*
  *Freshly ground pepper to taste*
- *2 tablespoons minced fresh Italian (flat-leaf) parsley*
- *5 pounds mussels, scrubbed, bearded, and rinsed*
- *8 ounces Swiss chard, well-rinsed and tough stems removed, finely chopped*
- *2 ripe plum tomatoes, diced*

1. Heat oil in a soup pot. Add shallots and garlic and cook over low heat, stirring, for 1 minute or until softened.

2. Add wine, bay leaf, thyme, pepper, and parsley to pot and bring to a boil. Let boil for 1 minute, then add mussels and stir. Using a slotted spoon, remove mussels as soon as they open, about 5 minutes, and

keep warm in a large serving bowl or deep platter. Discard any unopened mussels.

3. Add chard and tomatoes to liquid in pot and continue to boil, stirring occasionally, until liquid is reduced by half and chard is well-wilted. Discard bay leaf. Spoon chard and sauce over mussels and serve immediately.

SERVES 4

Per serving: 190 calories; 13.5 grams protein; 21.5 grams carbohydrates; 5.8 grams fat (2.1 grams fat from fish); 26 milligrams cholesterol; 400 milligrams sodium (without salting).

# STEAMED MUSSELS
# WITH PARSLEY PUREE

I wade right into eating these mussels by using a
fork to extract the first one from its shell. Then I
use the empty shell as tongs for getting the ivory-
white or amber-colored meat from the remaining
mussels. The exquisite juice, which mingles with
the verdant parsley sauce at the bottom of the bowl
is a reward—serve plenty of crusty country bread
to sop it up.

*2 cups packed fresh Italian parsley leaves*
*1 tablespoon olive oil*
*3 tablespoons dry vermouth*
   *Salt and freshly ground black pepper to taste*
*5 dozen mussels, scrubbed, bearded, and rinsed*
*1 cup Fish Stock (page 5) or canned low sodium broth*

1. Combine parsley, oil, vermouth, and salt and
pepper in a food processor and puree. Transfer to a
small bowl and reserve.

2. Combine mussels and fish stock in a large pot.
Cover tightly and steam over medium-high heat for
4 to 6 minutes, or until shells have opened. Discard
any mussels that have not opened.

3. Add parsley puree to mussels in pot and heat
through, uncovered, stirring to blend well. Transfer
mussels with its sauce to heated bowls and serve
hot.

Per serving: 130 calories; 12.5 grams protein; 6.5 grams carbohydrates; 6.0 grams fat (2.1 grams fat from fish); 26 milligrams cholesterol; 300 milligrams sodium (without salting).

# STEAMED LOBSTER WITH MUSHROOMS AND FETTUCCINE

I prefer the heavier live lobsters for this elegant dish, preferably the kind available from fall through early summer. If your market doesn't stock them, don't hesitate to use frozen Australian lobster tails which, though expensive, are not nearly as costly as the live, late-summer lobster that will deliver a forkful of meat and a pail full of water.

2 lobsters, 1½ to 2 pounds each
  Olive oil cooking spray
1 teaspoon olive oil
1 clove garlic, pressed
½ pound mushrooms, wiped clean and thinly sliced
½ cup Low Fat Chicken Stock (page 3) or canned low sodium broth
6 plum tomatoes, diced
  Salt and freshly ground pepper to taste
¾ pound fettuccine, cooked al dente
2 tablespoons minced fresh chives or scallions

1. Place lobsters in a very large pot and add about 3 inches of water. Cover, and bring to a boil over high heat. Steam for about 15 minutes or until lobsters are bright red and cooked through. Remove lobsters from pot and set aside to cool.

2. While lobsters cool, coat a large skillet with cooking spray. Add oil and heat. Add garlic and cook, stirring, for 1 minute. Add mushrooms and stock. Cover and cook over low heat for 4 to 5 minutes or until mushrooms have released their liquid. Add tomatoes and cook an additional 3 minutes. Remove skillet from heat.

3. Split lobsters and remove meat from body and claws. Cut meat into 1-inch pieces. Add lobster meat to skillet and put over very low heat, uncovered, until just warmed through. Don't let sauce boil as this will toughen the lobster. Season to taste with salt and pepper.

4. Place hot fettuccine in a mound in the center of a heated platter or individual dinner plates. Top noodles with lobster and sauce from skillet. Garnish with chives or scallions and serve.

SERVES 6

Per serving: 160 calories; 13.0 grams protein; 21.5 grams carbohydrates; 2.6 grams fat (.5 gram fat from fish); 50 milligrams cholesterol; 75 milligrams sodium (without salting).

# LIGHT QUENELLES DE POISSON

I've made these heavenly, light fish dumplings lighter still by using egg substitute instead of egg yolks, and by adding a minuscule amount of half-and-half with flour to replace the richness (and thickness) lost by omitting butter and cream. Finally, by using a sauce you could die for (Light Rouille or Almost Aioli) instead of the classic, rich white sauce you could die *from*, my Light Quenelles de Poisson becomes a dish you can live with indeed. Excellent as a light lunch.

4 cups Fish Stock (page 5)
1 1/2 pounds carp or whitefish fillets (or combination)
2 medium onions, quartered
   Egg substitute equal to 2 eggs, or 2 beaten eggs
   Salt and freshly ground pepper (preferably white) to taste
1/2 cup bread crumbs, made from 1 slice dry firm white bread
2 tablespoons flour
2 tablespoons half-and-half
1/2 cup Light Rouille (page 6) or Almost Aioli (page 7)

1. Bring stock to a simmer in a covered soup pot.
2. Cut fish into chunks and place in food processor with all remaining ingredients, except half-and-half and Light Rouille. Add half-and-half gradually, pro-

cessing until mixture is completely smooth. Transfer mixture to a medium bowl.

3. Using two tablespoons, form fish mixture into rounded ovals, approximately 2 inches long.

4. Keeping stock at a simmer, gently add fish ovals to pot. Cover and simmer for 30 minutes.

5. Using a slotted spoon, remove fish from stock and place in a deep bowl. Spoon stock around fish ovals so that they are almost covered with liquid. Refrigerate until chilled. Arrange quenelles on a platter or individual plates and serve with Light Rouille or Almost Aioli sauce on the side.

SERVES 4

Per serving: 320 calories; 32.0 grams protein; 22.0 grams carbohydrates; 11.0 grams fat (8.0 grams fat from fish); 96 milligrams cholesterol; 230 milligrams sodium (without salting).

# RED SNAPPER TORTILLAS

Here's a fish dish even the kids will eat with relish—or, more accurately, with salsa. And because the onions, salsa, and fish are cooked in the same skillet, it is quick, easy, and neat to prepare. The bonus is it's a healthy, fun *fin*-ger food the whole family can enjoy.

1½ pounds red snapper fillets
    Vegetable oil cooking spray
 1 small onion, diced
1½ cups Salsa Mexicana (page 8)
 8 corn tortillas, warmed
 1 cup packed shredded lettuce

1. Pour water into the bottom of a steamer. Place fish on steaming rack and cover. Bring water to a boil and steam for about 6 minutes or until fish flakes when tested with a fork. Remove fish from steamer and chop coarsely.

2. Coat a large nonstick skillet with cooking spray. Add onion and cook, stirring, for about 2 minutes or until onion is softened.

3. Add salsa to skillet and bring to a simmer. Add fish and simmer, uncovered, over medium heat briefly, until ingredients are just heated through.

4. Spoon 1 to 2 tablespoons of fish-salsa mixture in the center of a tortilla. Add 1 tablespoon of shred-

ded lettuce. Fold tortilla in half. Repeat with remaining tortillas, fish mixture, and lettuce.

SERVES 4
Per serving: 300 calories; 38.5 grams protein; 28.0 grams carbohydrates; 3.4 grams fat (2.3 grams fat from fish); 63 milligrams cholesterol; 145 milligrams sodium (without salting).

# BACK BAY SCROD HASH

Cod is a favorite along the cobbled streets of Boston, which both the upper-crust Brahman and the Boston Commoners treasure. Unfortunately, however, because of overfishing cod may soon be extinct. Just enjoy it while you can.

This divine combination of scrod, onion, and potatoes comes together when herbed stock is added to the mix. The hash then gets crisped under the broiler until golden brown. Serve it for breakfast, lunch, or dinner.

1 pound scrod or cod fillets
1 medium onion, quartered
4 medium potatoes, peeled and boiled
1/2 cup Low Fat Chicken Stock (page 3) or canned low sodium broth
2 tablespoons finely chopped fresh parsley
1/2 teaspoon freshly ground white pepper
1 teaspoon dried thyme
Salt to taste
Olive oil cooking spray

1. Preheat broiler to high.
2. Pour water into the bottom of a steamer. Place fish on steaming rack and cover. Bring water to a boil and steam for about 5 minutes, or until fish flakes when tested with a fork. Remove fish from steamer and let cool slightly.

3. Cut fish into chunks and place in food processor with onion. Process very briefly, until ingredients are just coarsely chopped.

4. Combine potatoes and stock in a large bowl and mash with a fork or a food mill. Add parsley, pepper, thyme, salt, and fish mixture to potatoes. Mix until ingredients are thoroughly combined.

5. Coat a nonstick baking pan with cooking spray. Spoon hash into bottom of pan and coat top with cooking spray. Do not smooth top; an uneven surface will result in crustier hash. Place pan 5 to 6 inches from heat and broil for 10 to 15 minutes, or until surface is browned and crisp. Serve hot.

SERVES 4

Per serving: 205 calories; 23.0 grams protein; 25.0 grams carbohydrates; 1.7 grams fat (.8 gram fat from fish); 49 milligrams cholesterol; 80 milligrams sodium (without salting).

# CHILLED POACHED SEA BASS

When poached, black bass is without peer for tenderness and moistness. And when poached in stock flavored with aromatic vegetables, it becomes a paradigm of pure taste.

This can be made a day or two in advance, covered and refrigerated. Serve the chilled bass either over or in the center of garnishes of your choice (cucumbers, scallions, endive, radishes, tomatoes, watercress, etc.) with the sauce on the side.

3 cups Fish Stock (page 5) or Low Fat Chicken Stock
    (page 3) or canned low sodium broth
1 cup dry white wine
1 carrot, thinly sliced
1 onion, quartered
4 sprigs fresh Italian parsley
    Salt and freshly ground pepper to taste
1 pound sea bass fillet, preferably in 1 piece
1 lemon, thinly sliced
1 cup Green Sauce with Shallots (page 10) or
    Cucumber Sauce (page 9)


1. Combine stock, wine, carrot, onion, and parsley in a soup pot and bring to a boil. Reduce heat, season to taste with salt and pepper and simmer for 15 minutes.

2. Add sea bass to liquid in pot. Cover and simmer gently for 5 to 8 minutes or until fish is just cooked

through. Using a slotted spatula, carefully transfer fish to a shallow dish, cover with lemon slices and spoon on enough cooking liquid to barely cover fish. Cool slightly, then cover and refrigerate for at least 2 hours.

3. Transfer chilled fish to a large platter and serve with Green Sauce with Shallots or Cucumber Sauce on the side.

SERVES 4

Per serving: 215 calories; 23.0 grams protein; 17.0 grams carbohydrates; 6.2 grams fat (2.3 grams fat from fish); 47 milligrams cholesterol; 150 milligrams sodium (without salting).

# POACHED SALMON STEAKS
# WITH CHILI CORN

One of the finest foods I know, and a great personal favorite, is poached salmon steaks. It also happens to be one of the simplest to prepare. The delicious chili corn is made by quickly heating the kernels and adding a judicious amount of chili powder—hot or mild, depending on your taste.

This makes a marvelous luncheon or supper dish, needing only a well-chilled bottle of dry white wine, a tossed salad, and an uncomplicated dessert.

  4 salmon steaks, about 5 ounces each
  4 tablespoons white wine vinegar
  1 large onion, sliced
  1 clove garlic
  4 sprigs fresh parsley and 4 sprigs dill tied together
  1/4 teaspoon white peppercorns
    Salt to taste
  2 teaspoons vegetable oil
  1/2 cup fresh or frozen and thawed corn
  1 teaspoon chili powder or to taste
  1 large lime cut into 4 wedges

1. Place salmon steaks in a large skillet or Dutch oven that can hold fish in one layer. Add enough cold water to cover fish. Add vinegar, onion, garlic, herb combination, peppercorns, and salt. Cover and

bring to a boil, then lower heat to a simmer. Poach salmon for 5 to 6 minutes or until fish is cooked through.

2. Meanwhile, heat oil in a small saucepan and add corn and chili powder. Cook over very low heat, stirring frequently, until fish is ready.

3. Using a slotted spatula, transfer fish to a serving platter. Spoon chili corn over salmon and serve garnished with lime wedges.

SERVES 4

Per serving: 250 calories; 28.5 grams protein; 8.0 grams carbohydrates; 11.8 grams fat (9.0 grams fat from fish); 64 milligrams cholesterol; 75 milligrams sodium (without salting).

# FLOUNDER AND POTATO CAKES

Fish and potato cakes are a popular "leftover" dish. My version uses freshly steamed flounder and spices them up with Dijon mustard and Worcestershire sauce. The Remoulade Sauce adds a tasty final touch.

Serve as a luncheon or supper dish, with a mixed green salad on the side.

1 pound flounder fillets
3 medium potatoes, peeled and boiled
1 medium onion, minced
  Egg substitute equal to 2 eggs
1 tablespoon Dijon mustard
2 teaspoons Worcestershire sauce
1 tablespoon finely chopped fresh dill weed
1/4 cup all-purpose flour
  Salt and freshly ground pepper to taste
1 tablespoon vegetable oil
1/2 cup Remoulade Sauce (page 13), at room
    temperature

1. Pour water into the bottom of a steamer. Place fish on steaming rack and cover. Bring water to a boil and steam for 4 to 5 minutes, or until fish flakes when tested with a fork. Remove fish from steamer and allow to cool.

2. Combine potatoes and onion and mash with a fork or in a food mill. Place potato mixture in a large

bowl. Add egg substitute, mustard, Worcestershire, and dill. Mix thoroughly.

3. Flake cooked fish with a fork and add to potato mixture, mixing just to combine. Place in refrigerator and allow mixture to chill for at least 1 hour.

4. Shape fish mixture into 12 thick, flat cakes.

5. Combine flour with salt and pepper and spoon mixture onto a plate. Dip fish-potato cakes in flour, shaking off excess.

6. Heat oil in a large nonstick skillet. Add cakes and sauté until golden brown on both sides. Drain fish cakes on paper towels, transfer to a platter, and serve with Remoulade Sauce on the side.

SERVES 4

Per serving: 280 calories; 29.5 grams protein; 25.0 grams carbohydrates; 7.0 grams fat (1.4 grams fat from fish); 55 milligrams cholesterol; 370 milligrams sodium (without salting).

# SNAPPER POACHED IN HERBED CLAM SAUCE

Serve with linguine or other pasta and a small salad of mixed greens.

  2 teaspoons olive oil
  1 onion, diced
  1 stalk celery, diced
  1 clove garlic, minced
  1 cup dry red wine
  2 cups Low Fat Chicken Stock (page 3) or canned low
      sodium broth
  2 ripe tomatoes, finely chopped, with juice
  1/2 teaspoon dried thyme
  1/2 teaspoon dried marjoram
  1 tablespoon minced fresh parsley or basil
      Salt and freshly ground pepper to taste
  1/2 cup minced clams, fresh or canned and drained
  4 black pitted olives, thinly sliced
  1 pound red snapper fillets

1. Heat oil in a wide soup pot or deep skillet. Add onion, celery, and garlic and cook over low heat, stirring frequently, for 3 minutes. Do not let vegetables brown.

2. Add wine, stock, and tomatoes to pot. Stir over low heat for 1 minute. Add thyme, marjoram, parsley or basil, and salt and pepper to taste.

3. Add clams and olives to pot and stir to combine.

Raise heat and bring to a simmer. Add snapper, cover and simmer for about 5 minutes or until fish is cooked through.

4. Using a slotted spatula, carefully remove fish and place on a heated serving platter. Spoon sauce over fish and serve.

SERVES 4

Per serving: 210 calories; 27.5 grams protein; 12.5 grams carbohydrates; 5.3 grams fat (1.5 grams fat from fish); 50 milligrams cholesterol; 200 milligrams sodium (without salting).

# INDEX

# *Enjoy Good Living All Year Long.*

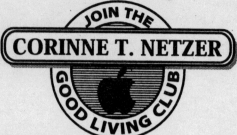

**JOIN THE**
## CORINNE T. NETZER
**GOOD LIVING CLUB**

Corinne T. Netzer, the country's foremost expert on good eating and good living, wants to share her wealth of knowledge with members of THE CORINNE T. NETZER GOOD LIVING CLUB. As a member, you'll receive *The Corinne T. Netzer Good Living Club Newsletter* twice a year. The newsletter will provide you with sound advice on any and every subject related to living well. Each issue will focus on a specific health-related subject and will provide information about current and upcoming Corinne T. Netzer books. Members will also receive information on special offers exclusive to THE CORINNE T. NETZER GOOD LIVING CLUB. What are you waiting for? Join today... and start living!

■